W9-DEU-291

a guide to

essential oils

a guide to essential oils

Jennie Harding

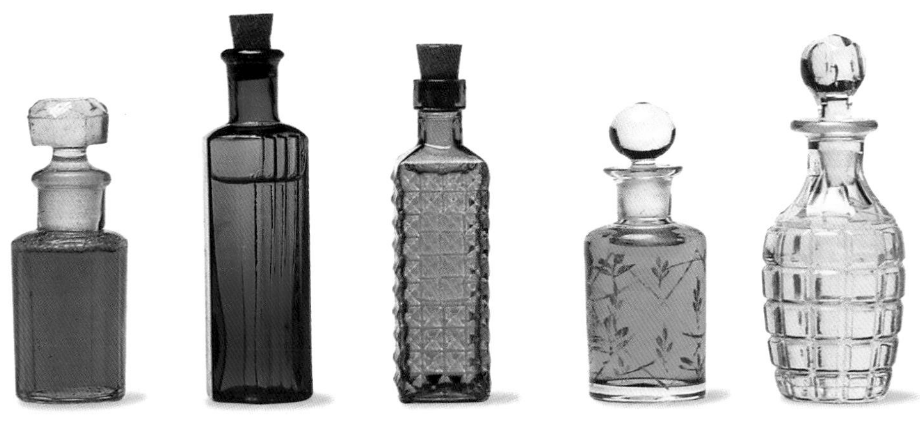

p

This is a Parragon Publishing Book
First published in 2002

Parragon Publishing
Queen Street House
4 Queen Street
Bath BA1 1HE, UK

ISBN: 0-75257-783-2

Printed in China.

Designed and created with the Bridgewater Book Company Ltd.

NOTE

Any information given in this book is not intended to be taken as a replacement for medical advice. Any person with a condition requiring medical attention should consult a qualified medical practitioner or therapist.

WARNING

Never leave a burning candle unattended.

ACKNOWLEDGMENTS

The publishers wish to thank the following for the use of pictures: *Art Directors and Trip*: 12t, 20b, 23t, 29t, 32t, 48t, 49b; *A–Z Botanical Collection Ltd*: 8b, 19t, 34t, 37t, 39t; *Corbis UK Ltd*: 18b, 23b, 38, 53t; *Garden Picture Library*: 47b; *Getty Images*: 7t, 10t, 11t, 24t, 36b, 59b; *Harry Smith Horticultural Photographic Collection*: 33t.

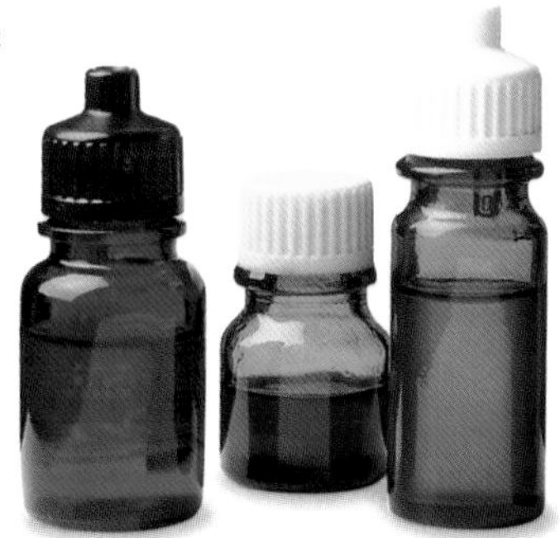

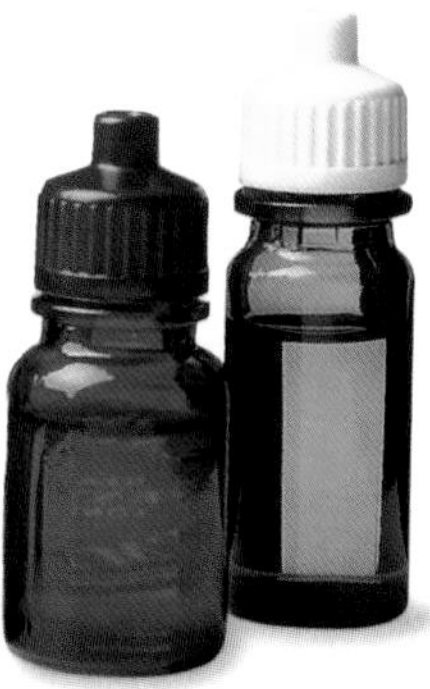

contents

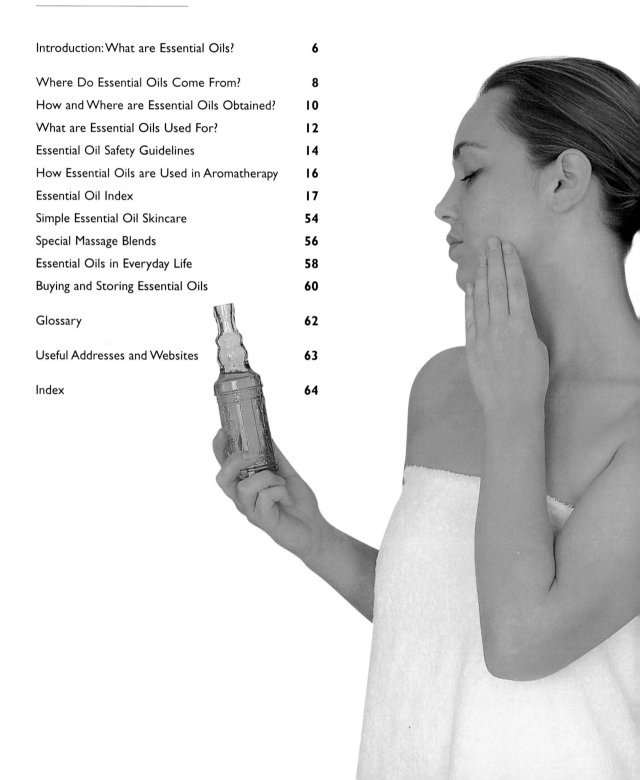

Introduction: What are Essential Oils?

Humans love aromatic plants. When we pass a beautiful, scented flower our behavior shows this very clearly. The fragrance is enough to stop us in our tracks, making us forget our train of thought and plunge our face into the petals to inhale the perfume. When we do, we forget the cares and troubles of the day for a moment, and the world seems to be a simpler place. Gardeners love to touch and smell the herbs and aromatic grasses that they grow themselves, sniffing the aromas that cling to the fingers, such as pungent rosemary or zesty peppermint, fresh lavender or tangy fennel. These mouthwatering scents make us relax and breathe deeply.

All these perfumes we are inhaling and enjoying so enthusiastically are essential oils, the natural fragrances of aromatic plants. These scents are manufactured by the plants themselves and held in their tissues, only to be released through touch or the heat of the sun. Of all the plants on the Earth, only about one percent contain essential oils. Humans have enjoyed a special relationship with these species since antiquity, and we have used such plants for perfumes, incense, and medicines.

The pungent herb rosemary uplifts the senses and excites the tastebuds. It is easily grown in a pot outside.

Aromatherapy relies on essential oils to achieve gentle, nurturing effects on body and mind. The oils are used on the skin, in the bath, and through inhalation to promote

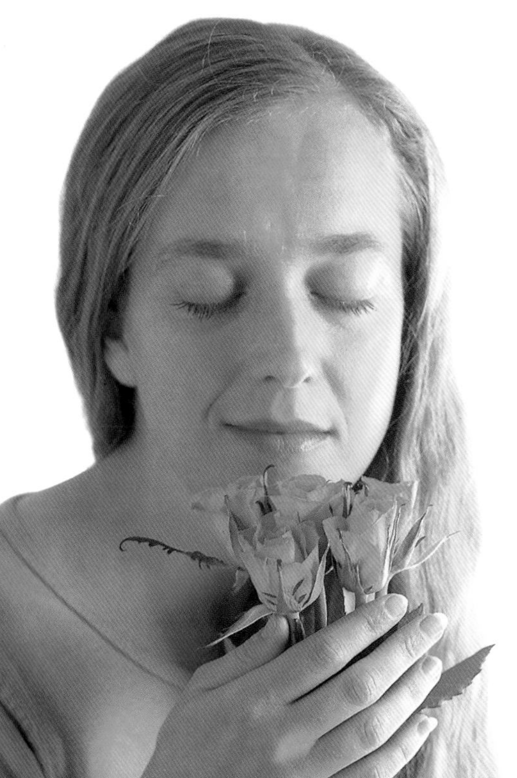

Flowers attract our sense of smell like a magnet. We are drawn to plants such as scented roses.

Relaxing in a bath with essential oils soothes the senses and can bring relief from aches and pains in the body.

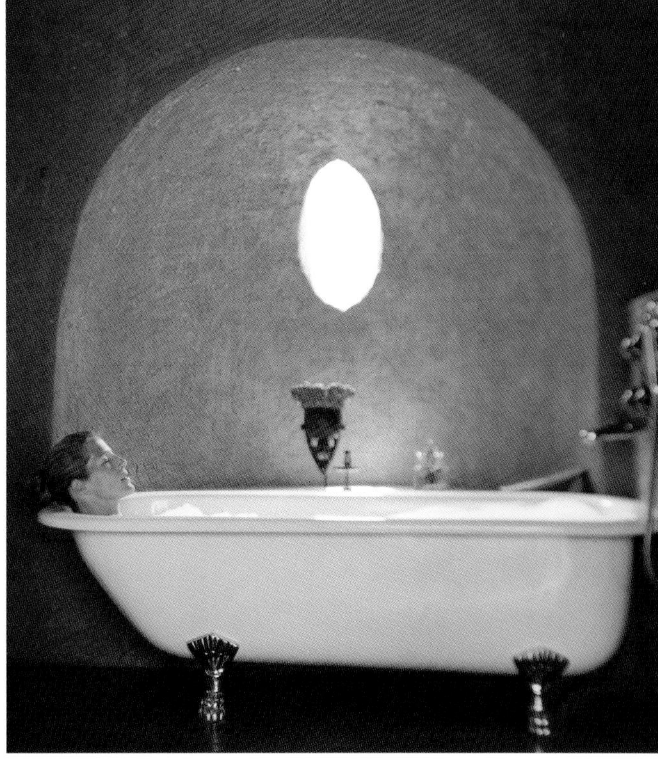

relaxation and well-being. Essential oils and aromatherapy can make a very positive contribution to emotional and physical health, bringing a sense of inner peace and balance.

The Guide to Essential Oils takes you on a journey through the world of essential oils, explaining where they come from and how they are obtained. It is an exploration of the particular plants that produce essential oils, revealing their unique role as a natural healing resource. The Essential Oils Index on pages 17–53 lists 36 common essential oils in detail, helping you get to know more about them and how to use them on yourself, friends, and family. The methods are straightforward and easy to use in everyday situations. You will also find information about safety issues, buying and keeping the oils, and simple skincare routines.

You may well find that collecting essential oils, enjoying their aromas, and learning about their different uses, becomes a fascinating pastime, something that develops from being a hobby into, quite simply, a way of life.

This book links the essential oils to the plants from which they are extracted. The botanical emphasis of this approach helps us to remember that all life on Earth is dependent on plants. As custodians of the planet, we need to use these natural resources in a sustainable way if we are to continue to enjoy them.

Peppercorns yield a warming and stimulating essential oil that can ease painful joints and muscles.

Where Do Essential Oils Come From?

Essential oils are obtained from a small variety of aromatic plants. To understand essential oils, it helps to know something about how plants that provide essential oils function: through their roots, wood, leaves, flowers, and fruits and seeds. Essential oils may be found in any of these plant parts.

Essential oils are found in a variety of plant parts. The roots, wood, leaves, flowers, and fruits and berries can all yield up their precious perfumes.

The Magic of Plants

Plants are the most amazing interactive energy systems, able to respond to the most minute changes in environmental conditions at all times during their life span. They are in the business of survival, competition, and reproduction, and over millions of years they have evolved precise mechanisms to achieve this, of which essential oils are one. Botanists are unsure why particular plants have evolved to contain essential oils. However, here are some suggestions.

Roots

Roots draw minerals and water into the plant tissue as well as giving stability to the growing plant. Aromatic roots such as turmeric or vetiver, which grow in hot tropical locations, are unsavory to invading grubs, beetles, and other insects. This helps to protect delicate root tissue from damage and promotes maximum water uptake.

Wood

Trees like sandalwood or cedarwood contain essential oils in the heartwood of their trunks

Essential oils in leaves may have a protective function. This is the ylang ylang plant—the beautiful blooms nestle within the large dark-green leaves and are protected from the elements.

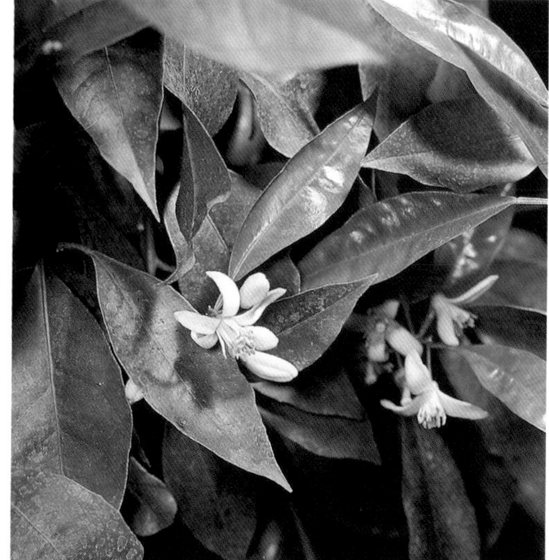

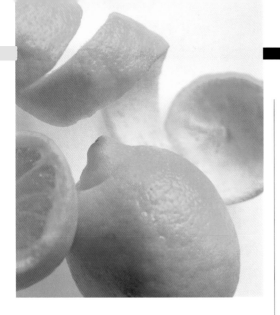

Essential oils that are found in the rind of fruits have a pungent and long-lasting aroma, making them popular scents.

and branches. There is some evidence that oils help to protect the inner structure of the wood from attack by beetles and other insects. Shrubs like frankincense and myrrh secrete resin, a sticky substance rich in essential oils, to protect themselves if their bark is cracked or damaged. The resin has been collected by humankind for thousands of years and burned as incense.

Leaves

In the leaves of any plant, the process of photosynthesis uses sunlight to convert carbon, hydrogen, and oxygen to sugars. This process is vital for the growth of the plant, its eventual flowering, and successful reproduction. Essential oils in the leaves may protect them from fungi or microbial attack, ensuring the maximum surface is available for the production of the plant's food.

Flowers

Some of the floral essential oils that are used in aromatherapy include subtle and exquisite fragrances such as lavender, rose, jasmine, or orange blossom. The essential oils of other plants, such as frangipani, tuberose, or mimosa, are very expensive to extract and are used in the formulation of some of the costliest perfumes. Flowers have only one purpose—to attract pollinating insects. The chemistry of attraction is a vital part of the insect–plant relationship. Some flowers have evolved aromas that mimic exactly the scent of specific insects. For example, the giant waterlily (*Victoria amazonica*) copies the pheremonal odor of a night-flying beetle that has been pollinating the plant for centuries. Humans also have a long tradition of using the aroma of flowers to attract a mate—hence our love of perfumes.

Fruits and Seeds

Essential oils can be extracted from the rind of all citrus fruits. They are also found in the berries of bushes such as juniper. Fruits and berries are the end result of the flowering process. They tend to be aromatic in order to encourage animals or birds to eat them. The seeds are indigestible and are therefore excreted into the soil, giving the seed a better chance of germinating successfully.

How and Where are Essential Oils Obtained?

The production of essential oils involves a considerable investment of time, labor, and skill. Plants are cultivated, harvested, and processed to produce oils, which may then be shipped vast distances before reaching the consumer. Essential oils are a natural resource dependent on correct balances of soil composition, sun, and rain to achieve good harvests year by year—just like any other natural crop.

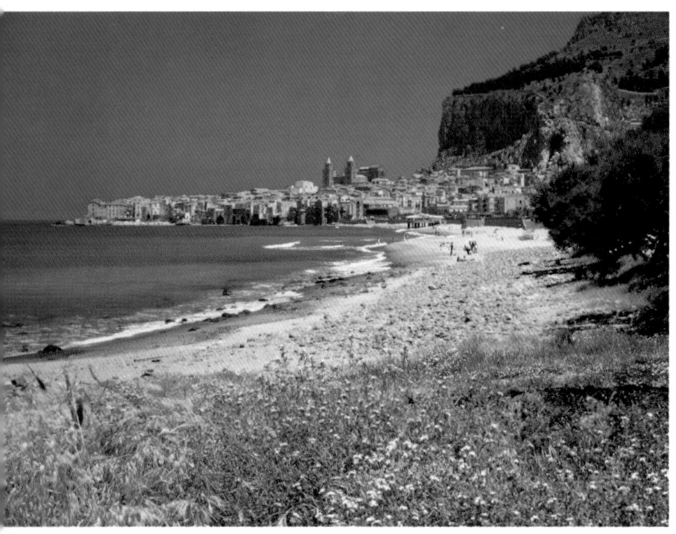

Many essential oils are found in distant locations world-wide. Mediterranean plants need sunlight to develop properly.

Geography

Essential oils are found in different plant groups all over the world. One of the most common is the botanical family *Labiatae,* which includes many Mediterranean plants such as rosemary, marjoram, and lavender. Most of the oils used in aromatherapy come from plants grown in southern Europe and North Africa, as these need a lot of sunlight to produce their oils. The same geographical region is the home of many citrus fruits in the *Rutaceae* family, including succulent oranges, lemons, and mandarins, whose peel is full of essential oil.

Farther afield you find the trees, flowers, and spices of India, for example, producer of jasmine, sandalwood, cardamom, and patchouli oils. Indonesia produces some of the more unusual oils, such as vetiver, which has a smoky, earthy aroma. The best geranium oil comes from the island of Réunion in the Indian Ocean, while Australia is the biggest producer of tea tree oil.

Cardamom pods produce a warm, fragrant, and spicy essential oil.

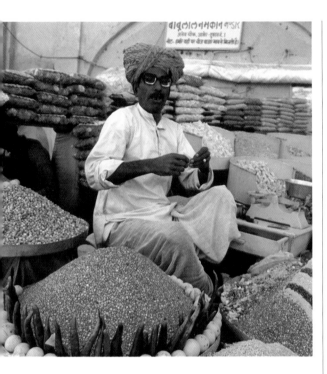

India is a huge producer of spices, aromatics, and fragrances. Some of the more unusual oils come from this great continent.

When buying an oil, check the Essential Oil Index (see pages 17–53) to see where it is produced and just how far it has traveled!

Cultivation

The cultivation of essential oils requires a lot of land to produce bulk supplies of plants. For example, it takes approximately half a tonne of lavender material to produce just 4 cups (1 liter) of essential oil. Successful lavender farms need many hectares of land.

Oils like vetiver are produced in developing countries where farmers use high levels of manual labor and traditional techniques. Very often the labor lies in the collection process where plants cannot be harvested mechanically. In Bulgaria, roses are picked off the bush by hand—roughly 50–100 rose blooms are used for one drop of essential oil.

More mechanized essential oil cultivation is found in Australia, where tea tree oil is produced on a large scale on plantations using modern machinery for harvesting.

Extraction Methods

Essential oils are held in sacs or special microscopic cells within the plant tissues themselves. To extract the oil, different techniques are used:

Steam distillation passes steam at high pressure through the plant material, releasing the globules of essential oil into the water vapor. The fragrant steam is cooled back to water, and the essential oil can then be skimmed off as it floats on the surface. This technique is used to extract most oils, including lavender and rosemary.

Expression involves pressing the oil directly out of citrus fruit peel.

Solvent extraction uses chemical solvents to dissolve aromatic compounds out of delicate plant tissues. The extract is refined to produce an "absolute." Jasmine oil is produced by solvent extraction.

What are Essential Oils Used For?

In the last ten years, more and more people have been using essential oils and aromatherapy has become very popular. However, it may surprise you to discover that essential oils have a long history of use, both in aromatherapy and in other areas.

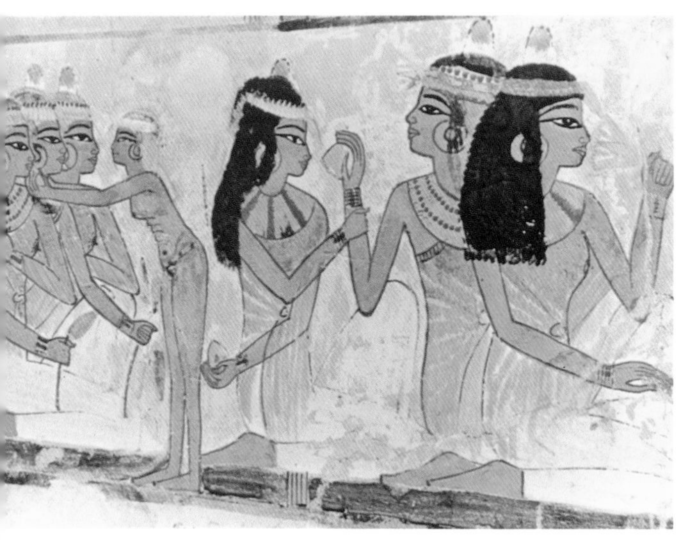

Ancient Egyptian men and women used aromatic fragrances to perfume the body and the hair.

Perfumery

Essential oils have been the basic ingredients in perfume formulae since the invention of a form of distillation by Avicenna, an Arab perfumer, mystic, and herbalist, at the beginning of the last millennium. Even before that, essential oils were extracted by a method called enfleurage, in which aromatic plant material was pressed into trays of fat, which were then heated in an oven or left out in the sun. The melted fat was strained and then left to set, and the solid, scented "unguent" used as a fragrance on the skin and hair.

In the past, only the most wealthy could afford the rare and costly extracts that were available. Perfumes were a sign of wealth and status. At the beginning of the twentieth century, the development of synthetic aromatic chemicals meant that perfume formulae could be copied, which is what happens in the mass production of fragrances today. Natural essential oils and aromatic extracts continue to be used for the creation of new formulae for perfumes, which are then synthetically reproduced.

Peppermint oil is used to flavor confectionery, including chocolates.

Food Flavoring

Many of the foodstuffs and drinks that we consume are flavored with essential oils. Obvious examples include the use of peppermint and citrus oils in chocolate and other confectionery. However, many oils are used to give "natural" flavors and fragrances to food products. They are used in preserved meats, alcoholic drinks, pickles, and sauces. The amounts of essential oil used are very small and are carefully monitored to be at safe levels for internal consumption, because essential oils are extremely concentrated. In aromatherapy, essential oils are never swallowed. (See "Essential Oil Safety Guidelines," pages 14–15.)

Pharmaceuticals

As well as being used in many foodstuffs, peppermint oil is used in pharmaceutical products such as toothpaste. Other essential oils that have pharmaceutical purposes include camphor and eucalyptus, which are used in commercial cough medicines, chest rubs, and ointments for muscular aches and pains. Many of these products have been licensed since the early twentieth century.

Aromatherapy

Of all the tonnes of essential oils produced world-wide each year, only about five to ten percent are used in aromatherapy. This is often a surprise to people, because they may be aware of essential oils only as the main ingredient in aromatherapy and not realize that they are so widely used elsewhere. In aromatherapy, it is very important that the oils used are totally natural and unadulterated with synthetics—trustworthy suppliers will buy directly from growers all around the world (for suppliers, see page 61).

Essential oils such as that found in the citrus fruit orange are often used as food flavorings and preservatives.

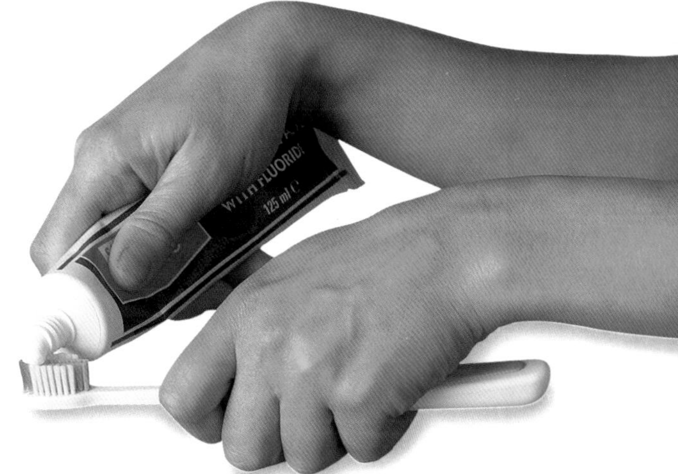

Essential oils such as peppermint or fennel are used to flavor different kinds of toothpaste the world over.

Essential Oil Safety Guidelines

Essential oils are completely natural. However, it is important to be aware that they are highly concentrated and need to be used safely and correctly. These guidelines will help you to check how to use essential oils in particular situations. It is advisable to consult your medical practitioner if you have any physical or psychological symptoms, as essential oils are not a replacement for professional medical treatment.

No to Oral Use

The most important safety guideline is simply this: do not take essential oils by mouth. They are highly concentrated substances and in large amounts they can do internal damage. If oils have been swallowed accidentally, seek medical help immediately.

Pregnancy Care

If you are pregnant, lactating, or breastfeeding, it is especially important not to swallow any essential oils. Any oils you use on yourself for massage or in the bath should be in very weak dilutions. If you are making any of the blends in this book, you should use half the stated number of drops. You are best advised to use flower and fruit oils only, as these are very gentle. It is a good idea to consult a qualified aromatherapist for advice.

Women who are pregnant or breastfeeding need to be very careful when using essential oils.

Skin Safety

Before being applied to the skin, essential oils should always be diluted in a carrier oil such as sweet almond or grapeseed because they are so concentrated. Provided that you do not have sensitive skin (a tendency to allergic reactions), you can use lavender or tea tree neat for first-aid purposes (two drops on a cotton swab applied to the affected area). If you are sensitive to nuts, it is best to avoid sweet almond oil and use grapeseed instead.

Phototoxic Oils

Essential oils from the citrus fruits—bergamot, grapefruit, orange, lemon, lime, and mandarin—contain an ingredient that can cause skin

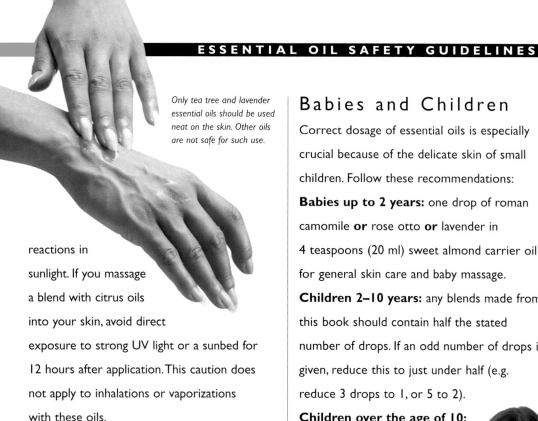

Only tea tree and lavender essential oils should be used neat on the skin. Other oils are not safe for such use.

reactions in sunlight. If you massage a blend with citrus oils into your skin, avoid direct exposure to strong UV light or a sunbed for 12 hours after application. This caution does not apply to inhalations or vaporizations with these oils.

High Blood Pressure

Rosemary essential oil is very stimulating and should be avoided if you have high blood pressure. Calming oils like lavender or ylang ylang are preferred for their soothing effects.

Epilepsy and Asthma

Again, rosemary essential oil has the potential to slightly increase the frequency of epileptic seizures, so it should be avoided by people with epilepsy. Calming oils like sandalwood, neroli, or orange are more appropriate. (Never attempt to apply oils during a seizure.) If you have asthma, it is advisable not to do inhalations with essential oils—use them for bathing, vaporization, and massage.

Babies and Children

Correct dosage of essential oils is especially crucial because of the delicate skin of small children. Follow these recommendations:

Babies up to 2 years: one drop of roman camomile **or** rose otto **or** lavender in 4 teaspoons (20 ml) sweet almond carrier oil for general skin care and baby massage.

Children 2–10 years: any blends made from this book should contain half the stated number of drops. If an odd number of drops is given, reduce this to just under half (e.g. reduce 3 drops to 1, or 5 to 2).

Children over the age of 10: can receive oils in the same dilutions as adults.

Elderly Skin

In cases where the skin is delicate and very transparent with visible veins, you should use half the stated number of drops in any blend you make from this book so that the skin is nourished by the oils more gently.

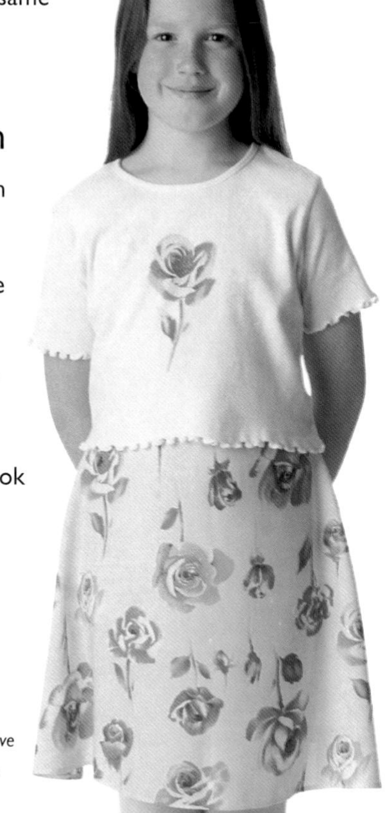

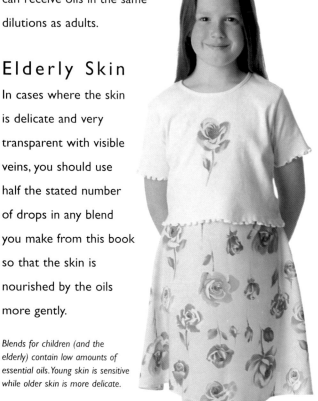

Blends for children (and the elderly) contain low amounts of essential oils. Young skin is sensitive while older skin is more delicate.

How Essential Oils are Used in Aromatherapy

Aromatherapy is what it says it is—the "aroma" being the fragrances of essential oils, and the "therapy" the way in which the fragrance is applied to relieve physical symptoms and promote mental well-being. There are several simple ways to use essential oils, including in baths, inhalation, and massage.

Baths

For a 20-minute soak to relieve tension and stress, run the bath to a comfortable temperature. Sprinkle 4 drops maximum of one essential oil or 3 drops each of two essential oils as a combination onto the surface of the water. Agitate the water gently to disperse the oils before getting in. If you have dry or sensitive skin, you can dilute the essential oils in 4 teaspoons (20 ml) whole milk or unfragranced bath oil before adding to the water. A relaxing combination is 3 drops each of lavender and sandalwood.

Inhalation

This method helps to relieve colds, influenza, or sinus problems. You need a large bowl just over half full of nearly boiling water. Sprinkle 2 drops each of eucalyptus and tea tree onto the surface, then cover your head with a towel and inhale the aromatic steam for 15–20 minutes. Remove your glasses or contact lenses so they don't steam up or irritate the eyes.

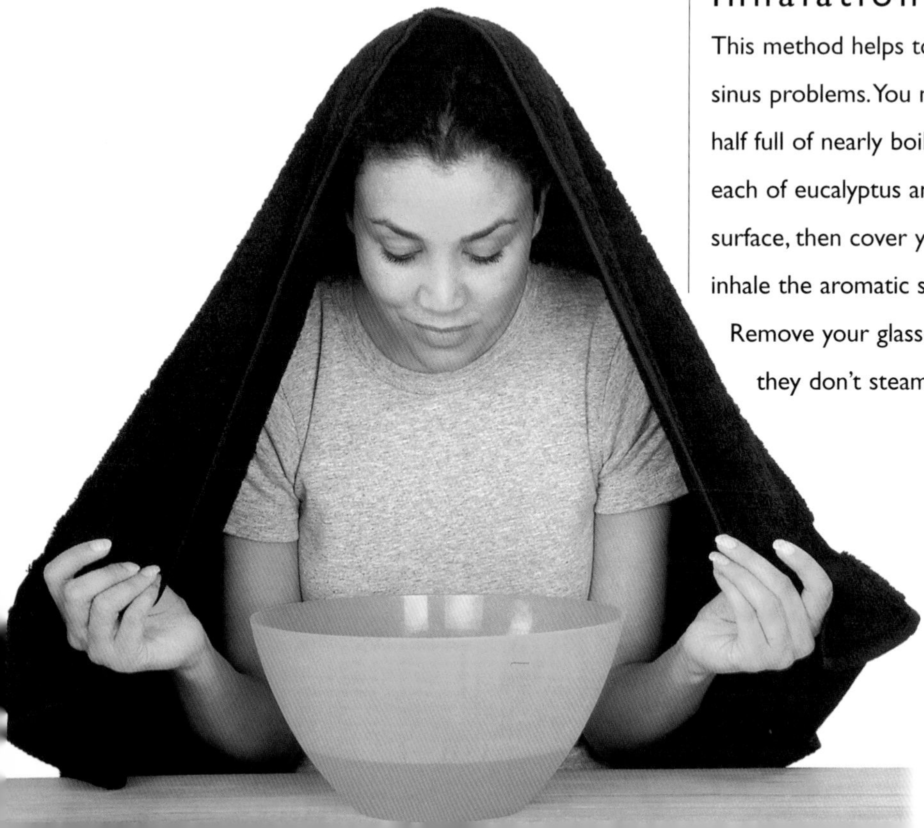

Using steam inhalation can help to ease colds or blocked sinuses. Always be very careful when using boiling water.

Vaporization

Vaporizers gently heat up to evaporate the essential oil and disperse its fragrance into a room. You can buy a ceramic burner with tea light candles or one of the many electric models available. You should follow the manufacturer's guidelines when using the oils though; generally 4 drops of one oil or 3 drops each of two as a combination will scent a room for up to two hours. You can use tea tree and lemon essential oils to remove unpleasant odors, or choose a favorite aroma to create an environment that suits your mood.

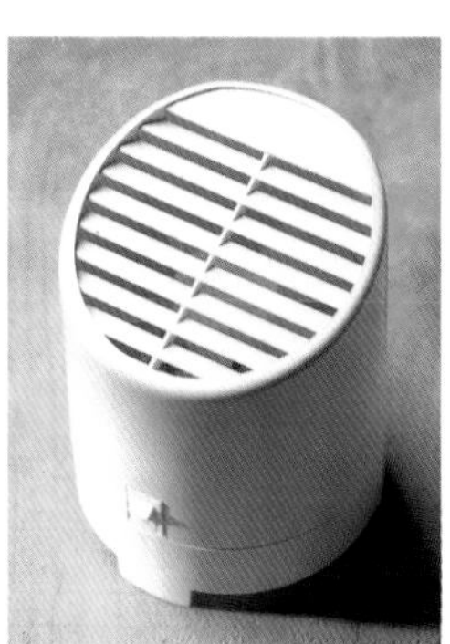

An electrically powered fragrance diffuser can help ease breathing problems and is safe to be left on.

Massage

When using essential oils for massage, they first need to be diluted in a carrier oil. These are vegetable oils such as grapeseed, sweet almond, or jojoba. Most of the massage blends in this book are based on a formula of using 10 drops of essential oils in 4 teaspoons (20 ml) carrier oil. The mixture should be stored in a clean glass bottle. Shake the mixture before use. This is a suitable dilution for massage on most skins and is enough to massage a full body, not including the face. Sensitive, very young, or elderly skin requires only 5 drops in 4 teaspoons (20 ml). (See pages 56–57 for Special Massage Blends.) Your blends will last for a maximum of four weeks. If you want to make larger quantities, simply take 8 teaspoons (40 ml) base oil and double the drops of essential oils in the blend formula.

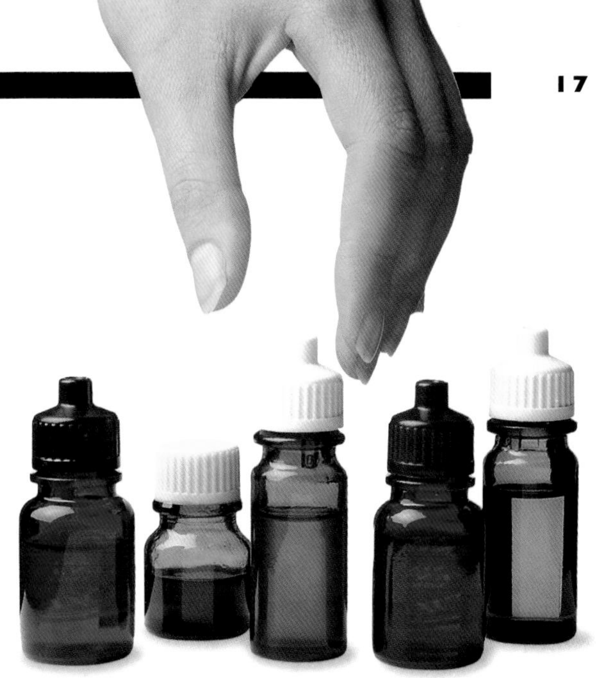

Choose the essential oil that meets your particular need, then blend with massage oil, bathe with it, or use in an inhalation.

Essential Oil Index

In this section, you will find 36 essential oils grouped according to the plant parts that produce them. Each essential oil file contains key information and blends to try out yourself to help ease physical conditions and rebalance mental and emotional states.

Root Oils

The energy of these oils is generally stabilizing and grounding to the body. Originally they protect and strengthen the plants that produce them.

Ginger

Zingiber officinale

Pungent ginger root yields a warming and spicy essential oil. It can improve energy levels.

Plant profile: ginger is a key ingredient in the recipes of India and China. It is also used in Traditional Chinese Medicine for digestion and circulation problems. Ginger roots are dried before distillation, which means that the essential oil smells less pungent than the freshly chopped root.

Safety information: no issues.

Fragrance profile: ginger has a dry, musty aroma, which is sharper and spicier as it evaporates, leaving behind a lingering sweetness.

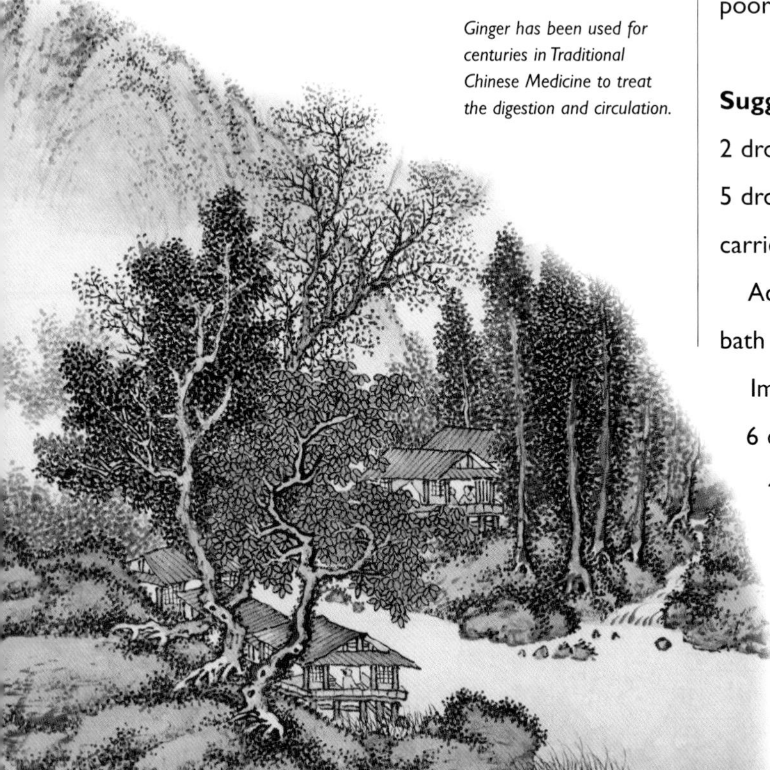

Ginger has been used for centuries in Traditional Chinese Medicine to treat the digestion and circulation.

Main uses: eases indigestion; warms and soothes aches and pains in muscles; improves poor circulation; improves energy.

Suggested blends: for indigestion, add 2 drops peppermint, 3 drops ginger, and 5 drops lemon to 4 teaspoons (20 ml) of carrier oil, then massage into the abdomen.

Aches and pains can be eased by taking a bath with 4 drops lavender and 2 drops ginger.

Improve circulation by massaging a blend of 6 drops black pepper and 4 drops ginger in 4 teaspoons (20 ml) carrier oil into the skin. You will notice the area becomes pink—this indicates improved circulation and is quite normal.

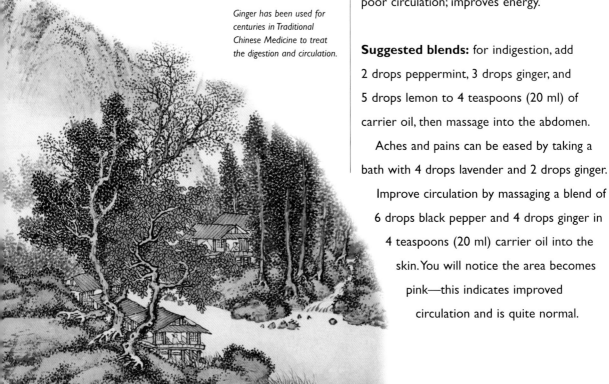

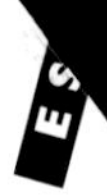

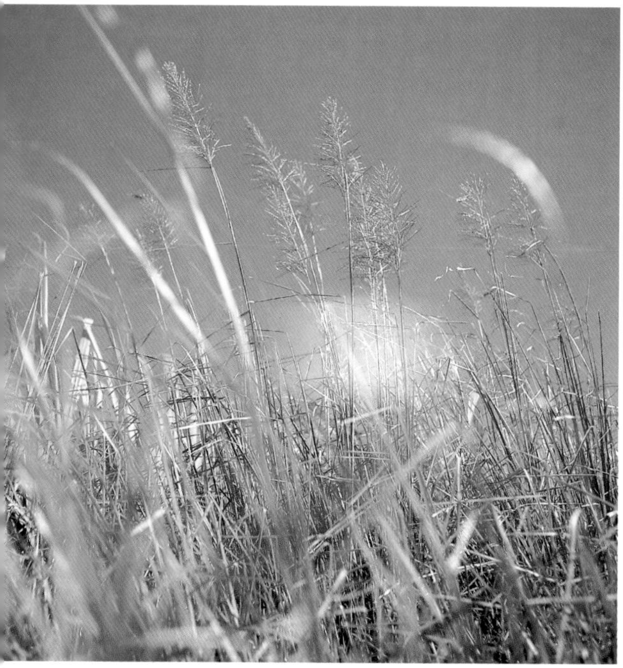

Vetiver

Vetiveria zizanoides

Plant profile: vetiver comes mainly from Indonesia, where it is known locally as *akar wangi*. It is a tough tropical grass that is economically important to growers. The upper leaves can be woven into mats and fibers, while the aromatic roots are harvested for distillation. Vetiver is also grown on the island of Réunion in the Indian Ocean.

Safety information: no issues.

Fragrance profile: a very unusual deep, earthy, smoky aroma, heavy and warm.

Vetiver is a very successful commercial c being a valuable essential oil.

Main uses: warms and re... pains, particularly backache; improves circulation; eases menstrual cramps; helps to ground and stabilize the emotions in cases of extreme stress.

Suggested blends: vetiver has a strong aroma, so use no more than 2 drops in a blend. For aches and pains and circulation, try 2 drops vetiver, 3 drops ginger, and 5 drops lavender in 4 teaspoons (20 ml) carrier oil for daily massage.

Ease menstrual cramps with a blend of 8 drops marjoram and 2 drops vetiver in 4 teaspoons (20 ml) carrier oil, massaged over the lower abdomen twice daily.

Emotional insecurity can be calmed by taking a bath with 1 drop vetiver, 1 drop neroli, and 3 drops lavender. Or add these oils to 2 teaspoons (10 ml) carrier oil and massage into the skin after your bath.

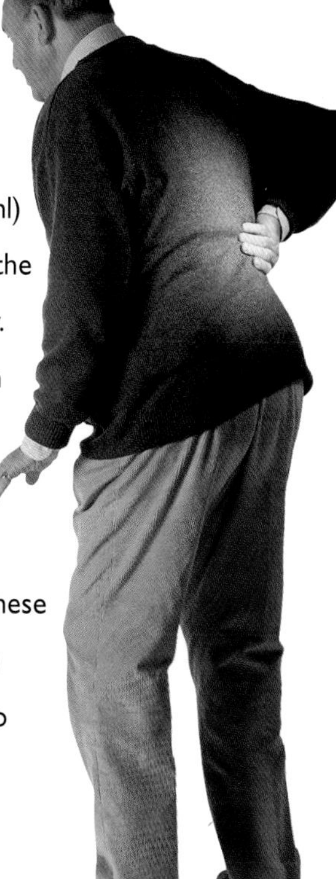

Massage an aching back with vetiver for relief from the pain. The warming scent is also very soothing to the mind and senses.

Angelica

Angelica archangelica

The whole of the angelica plant is aromatic. However, it is the root of the plant that is used in the distillation of the essential oil.

Plant profile: a herb that has been highly regarded in Western herbal tradition since medieval times, angelica is now cultivated for essential oil extraction in countries including Germany and Hungary. The whole plant is aromatic. It grows to about 6 feet (2 meters) high and has dramatic spherical heads of tiny flowers. The pungent root has been used in herbal medicine for hundreds of years as a general cleanser and detoxifier.

Safety information: angelica essential oil is phototoxic. After any application to the skin, avoid direct exposure to strong sunlight or a sunbed for 12 hours. Angelica oil is best avoided in pregnancy.

The angelica plant produces beautiful spherical flowerheads. These are made up of thousands of tiny flowers. Angelica is now specifically cultivated for essential oil extraction.

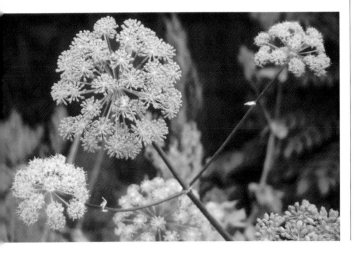

Fragrance profile: sweet and aniseed-like, with a rich, warm, and spicy note that is released as it evaporates.

Main uses: eases muscular aches, soothes arthritic joints and rheumatic pains; eases indigestion problems and wind and improves poor appetite; an overall energy tonic and revitalizer, especially in the springtime.

Suggested blends: for muscular aches and pains, add 2 drops angelica, 2 drops vetiver, and 5 drops lavender to 4 teaspoons (20 ml) carrier oil and apply using gentle massage.

Digestion problems can be eased by blending 3 drops peppermint, 4 drops ginger, and 3 drops angelica in 4 teaspoons (20 ml) carrier oil for massage over the abdomen.

A "springtime blend" to help to energize and tone body and mind is 2 drops angelica, 3 drops juniper, and 5 drops grapefruit in 4 teaspoons (20 ml) carrier oil, to be massaged into the skin after a bath or shower.

Turmeric

Curcuma longa/Curcuma domestica

Plant profile: turmeric is a plant that looks very like ginger, with tall shoots and abundant elegant leaves, and is a member of the same botanical family. The highly aromatic roots are bright yellow and are used to color curries. The roots are cleaned and sun-dried before being ground as a spice or distilled for the oil. India, China, and Indonesia are the main producers.

Safety information: no issues.

Fragrance profile: dry, musty, and vegetable-like aroma; spicy and sweet as it evaporates.

Main uses: soothes and eases backache and muscular pains; improves circulation; tones and improves the digestion, easing stomach cramps and constipation. Very stabilizing and grounding to overwrought emotions; warms and re-energizes the body.

Suggested blends: for aches and pains, add 4 drops turmeric, 4 drops ginger, and 2 drops vetiver to 4 teaspoons (20 ml) carrier oil and apply using gentle massage.

Yellow turmeric roots have many uses—they can be used as a cooking spice or an essential oil.

Cramps and indigestion can be eased by blending 4 drops turmeric, 2 drops lemongrass, and 4 drops ginger in 4 teaspoons (20 ml) carrier oil, then massaging the blend into the abdomen.

For emotional tension, add 1 drop turmeric, 2 drops neroli, and 2 drops ginger to a warm bath and rest there for 20 minutes. This can also be added to 2 teaspoons (10 ml) carrier oil and massaged into the skin afterward.

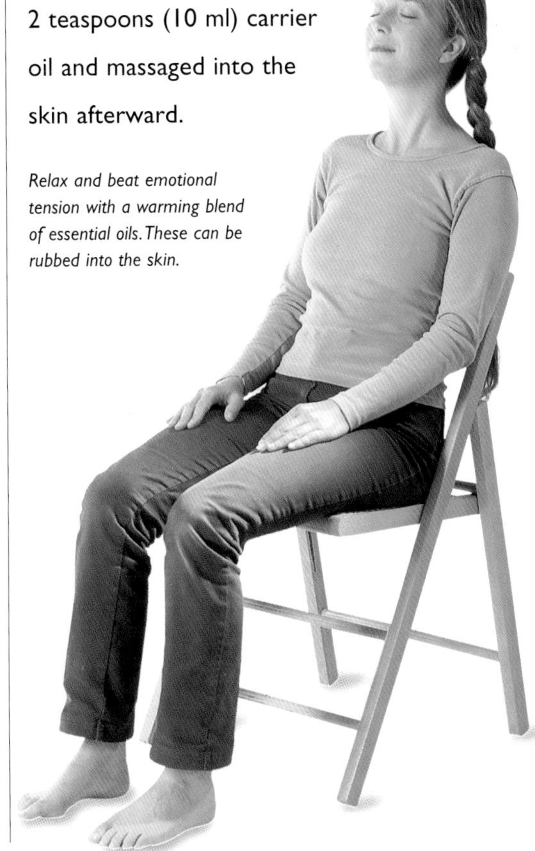

Relax and beat emotional tension with a warming blend of essential oils. These can be rubbed into the skin.

Wood Oils

These oils are found in the aromatic heartwood in the center of tree trunks and branches. They are at the core of the growing, spreading height of the tree. The energy of these oils is more expansive, encouraging deep breathing.

Sandalwood

Santalum album

Plant profile: the best-quality sandalwood comes from the Mysore region of India near Bangalore. It takes approximately 30 years for the wood to mature to its full aromatic potential, so planting and harvesting is carefully rotated and controlled. The wood is used in the distillation of sandalwood oil. It is also powdered for making incense sticks and cosmetics, and can be carved into statues and boxes.

Safety information: no issues.

Fragrance profile: this beautiful oil should be thick and pale golden, with a subtle aroma at first, deepening to a rich, woody, spicy, sweet fragrance as it evaporates.

Main uses: eases tight chesty coughs, colds, sore throats; soothes dry chapped skin and improves the texture of all skin types; eases depression, anxiety, and feelings of panic.

Suggested blends: for coughs, add 3 drops sandalwood, 3 drops cedarwood, and 4 drops lemon to 4 teaspoons (20 ml) carrier oil and massage gently over the chest area. A rejuvenating skincare blend is 6 drops sandalwood, 2 drops patchouli, and 2 drops rose in 4 teaspoons (20 ml) jojoba oil, massaged into the face at night. For anxiety or depression, add 3 drops sandalwood and 2 drops orange to a warm bath and rest for 20 minutes. Add the same oils to 2 teaspoons (10 ml) carrier oil and massage into the skin afterward.

Sandalwood brings a state of peace and calm to body and mind. It is also good for use on sensitive skins.

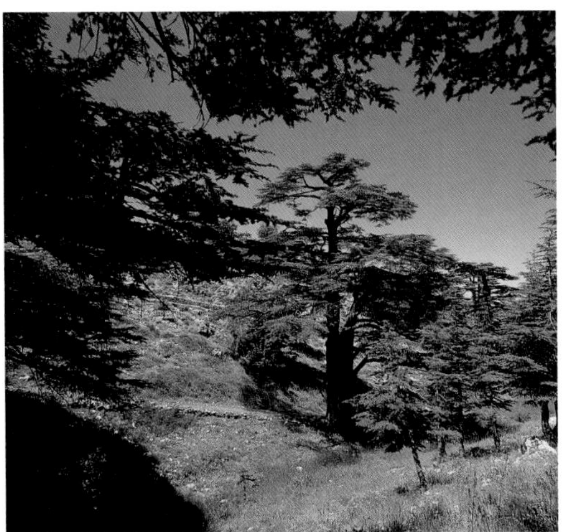

Cedarwood trees are huge and majestic, and are wonderfully aromatic too. The oil comes from the red heartwood.

Atlas Cedarwood

Cedrus atlantica

Plant profile: these tall, majestic cedar trees come from the Atlas mountains in Morocco. They stand over 100 feet (30 meters) in height with a sweeping, tentlike appearance, and a wonderful aroma floats around them thanks to the essential oil in the red heartwood. Cedar was used extensively by the ancient Egyptians in the manufacture of furniture and ships because of the wood's resistance to insects—as well as its beauty.

Safety information: no issues.

Fragrance profile: sharp and fresh with a sweet, woody, soft undertone.

Main uses: eases bronchitis, chest infections, coughs; soothes cracked skin, eczema, acne, and oily skin; assuages feelings of panic, calms and deepens the breath when under stress.

Suggested blends: Use 4 teaspoons (20 ml) carrier oil. For chest problems, add 3 drops cedarwood, 3 drops sandalwood, and 4 drops lemon and massage the chest. For cracked skin, add 3 drops cedarwood, 2 drops frankincense, and 5 drops lavender. For acne or oily skin, try 3 drops cedarwood, 2 drops tea tree, and 5 drops lavender in jojoba as a cleanser. For stress, vaporize 2 drops cedarwood and 3 drops lavender. Use these oils in 2 teaspoons (10 ml) carrier oil to massage the neck and shoulders.

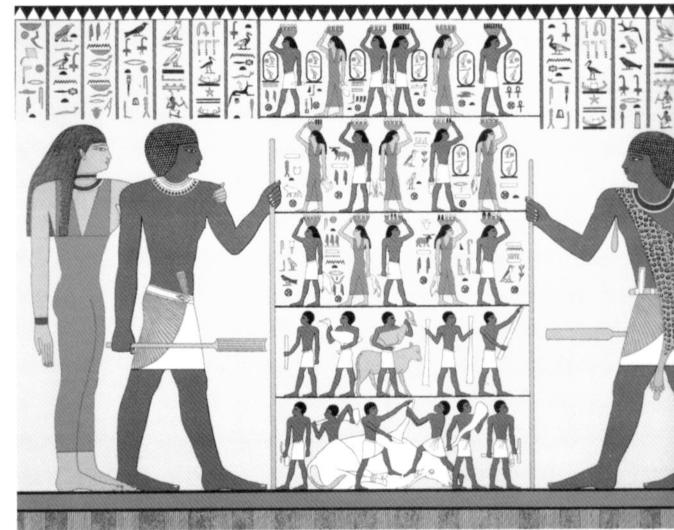

The ancient Egyptians used fragrant cedarwood to make beautiful and aromatic furniture.

Resin Oils

These sticky aromatic substances, the original incense ingredients, ooze out of the bark of certain trees and shrubs as a defense against injury. We too can use them to heal our skin.

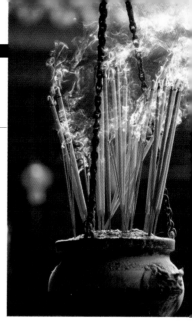

Frankincense

Boswellia carterii* var. *thurifera

Frankincense is the original "true incense" of antiquity and has been burned in places of religious worship for centuries.

Plant profile: frankincense is a robust desert shrub with delicate leaves and whitish papery bark. The name actually means "true incense," and it has been burned in religious ceremonies since ancient times. The frankincense plantations of the pharaohs were seen as one of the most valuable commodities in Egypt and frankincense was used in the embalming process. Cuts were made in the bark to make the gum ooze out. It is still used for incense and distilled for the oil, mainly in Somalia and Oman.

Safety information: no issues.

Frankincense gum forms "tears" or granules. This oozes out of the bark of the frankincense shrub when it is cut.

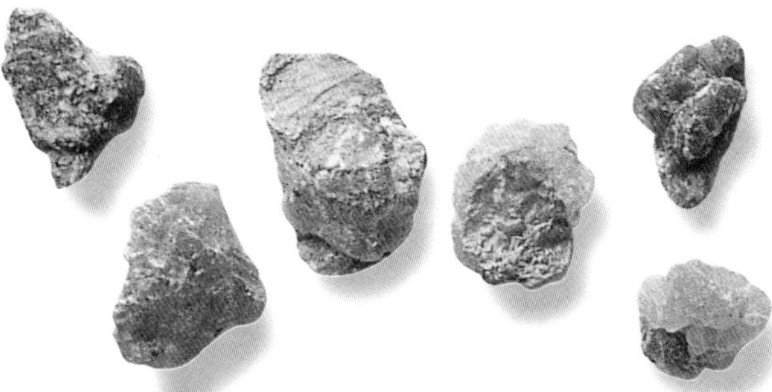

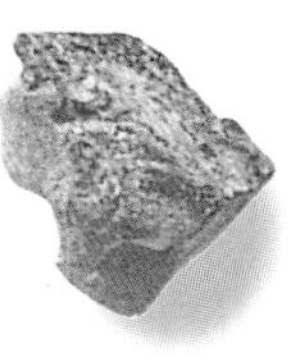

Fragrance profile: fresh and sharp initially, deepening to woody, resiny with sweet notes.

Main uses: disinfects and heals cuts, wounds, eczema, and damaged skin; tones and rejuvenates all skin types, especially mature; eases chesty coughs or bronchitis; comforts anxiety and emotional stress.

Suggested blends: a good skin-healing blend is 4 drops frankincense, 2 drops lavender, and 4 drops cedarwood in 4 teaspoons (20 ml) carrier oil. Apply twice daily. A tonic for mature skin is 4 drops frankincense, 3 drops neroli, and 3 drops rose in 4 teaspoons (20 ml) jojoba oil. For chesty coughs, try an inhalation of 3 drops frankincense and 3 drops cedarwood. To ease emotional stress and help you relax, vaporize 3 drops frankincense and 4 drops grapefruit.

Myrrh

Commiphora myrrha

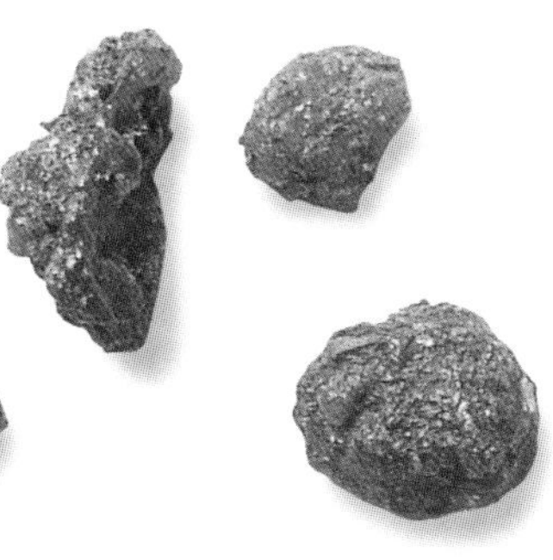

Myrrh gum is reddish-orange in color and was used in the embalming process in ancient Egypt.

Plant profile: a thorny shrub, native to the arid climates of Somalia and Arabia, with papery bark and a reddish gum that oozes out when the bark is cracked or cut deliberately. Myrrh is soluble in water and has been used as a tonic for the teeth and gums since the time of Hippocrates (469–399 BCE), the father of Western medicine. Like frankincense, myrrh is prized for wound healing, and was used by the ancient Egyptians for embalming.

Safety information: myrrh is best avoided during pregnancy.

Fragrance profile: a dry, sharp, and subtle aroma, which gradually deepens to reveal rich, sweet, and spicy notes.

Main uses: heals and disinfects deep cuts, wounds, chapped and cracked skin, eczema; cleans and disinfects the mouth, easing sore gums and mouth ulcers; relieves bronchitis, chesty coughs; comforts and calms highly anxious emotional states.

Suggested blends: Use 4 teaspoons (20 ml) carrier oil. To help damaged skin, add 3 drops myrrh, 4 drops tea tree, and 3 drops frankincense and apply 2–3 times daily. For chesty coughs, add 3 drops myrrh, 3 drops frankincense, and 4 drops cedarwood and massage the chest area, especially at night. For problems in the mouth, add 2 drops myrrh to a glass of water, then stir vigorously and use as a mouthwash (do not swallow). To de-stress, add 2 drops myrrh and 3 drops geranium to a bath—and relax.

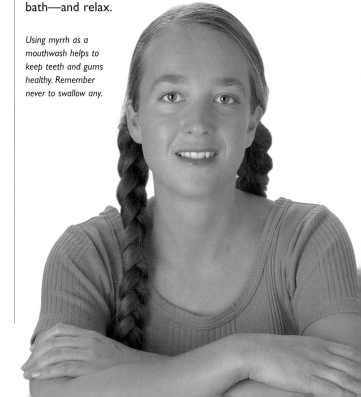

Using myrrh as a mouthwash helps to keep teeth and gums healthy. Remember never to swallow any.

Leaf Oils

These oils are contained in the all-important leaves that manufacture the plant's food. They protect the leaf surface from damage by fungi and bacteria.

Marjoram

Origanum marjorana

Plant profile: this is the species otherwise known as "French marjoram," and not Spanish marjoram, which is a type of thyme. French marjoram has been a favorite herb for cooking and has been widely used for centuries. It is low-growing, with small aromatic leaves and tiny white flowers that appear in summer. Originally from Mediterranean regions, it will grow well in more northerly climates if kept sheltered and in a sunny spot. The essential oil comes from France.

Safety information: no issues.

Fragrance profile: a warm, woody aroma that somewhat resembles camphor, gradually becoming sweet and soft.

French marjoram has a gentle woody aroma. The scent evaporates quite quickly.

Main uses: helps muscular aches and pains, stiffness, and strains; eases menstrual cramps and mood swings; helps migraine, headaches, and nervous tension.

Suggested blends: Use 4 teaspoons (20 ml) carrier oil. For muscular aches, add 4 drops marjoram, 4 drops ginger, and 2 drops vetiver for massage. For menstrual symptoms, add 4 drops marjoram, 4 drops lavender, and 2 drops vetiver, then massage the abdomen.

For headaches and nervous tension, add 4 drops marjoram, 2 drops peppermint, and 4 drops lavender and then gently massage the forehead, neck, and shoulders.

Using essential oils like marjoram can help headaches and menstrual problems.

Peppermint

Mentha piperita

Peppermint is a scented herb a very easily an the garden.

Plant profile: peppermint is a tall vigorous mint with a very invasive habit—ask any gardener! It spreads rapidly through tough root systems, and will displace other more tender herbs in a plot unless it is contained in some way. The square, erect stems support deep-green aromatic leaves and, if left untrimmed, the plant will produce tall heads of tiny white flowers. Peppermint essential oil comes mostly from the USA, and is used, in particular, to flavor toothpaste and chewing gum.

Safety information: if your skin is sensitive, use half the stated drops of peppermint in any blend due to the menthol content in the oil, which can act as an irritant.

Fragrance profile: pungent, fresh, zesty, and minty aroma with sweeter notes later.

Main uses: eases stomach cramps, indigestion, constipation, and nausea; helps muscular aches, stiffness, backache; eases headaches and migraine; clears the head and improves concentration.

Suggested blends: Use 4 teaspoons (20 ml) carrier oil. For indigestion symptoms, add 2 drops peppermint, 4 drops ginger, and 4 drops cardamom and massage the abdomen.

For aches and pains, add 2 drops peppermint, 4 drops rosemary, and 4 drops black pepper, and massage daily. To ease headaches, add 2 drops peppermint and 3 drops lavender to 2 teaspoons (10 ml) carrier oil and massage onto the forehead and neck.

For clearing the mind, vaporize 2 drops peppermint and 3 drops lemon.

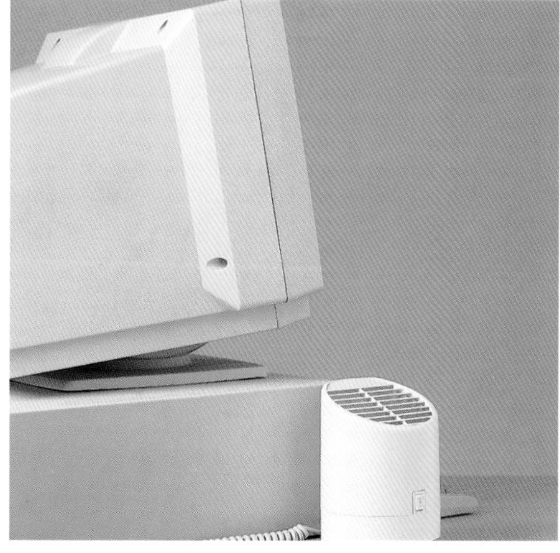

Vaporizing peppermint essential oil in the office can clear your head and kick-start the mind.

Rosemary

Rosmarinus officinalis

Rosemary is an evergreen herb with a bracing aroma. It is used in cooking as well as aromatherapy.

Plant profile: the name "rosemary" means "rose of the sea," a reference to the original habitat of the plant on the dry, sandy coastline of the Mediterranean Sea. Even today, the best pungent oil comes from Spain or North Africa; the hotter and dryer the climate, the better the aroma. Rosemary oil smells quite similar to eucalyptus because they have a fragrant ingredient in common: eucalyptol.

Safety information: rosemary is not advised for people with high blood pressure, as it is a stimulating oil. It should also be avoided by people who suffer from epilepsy.

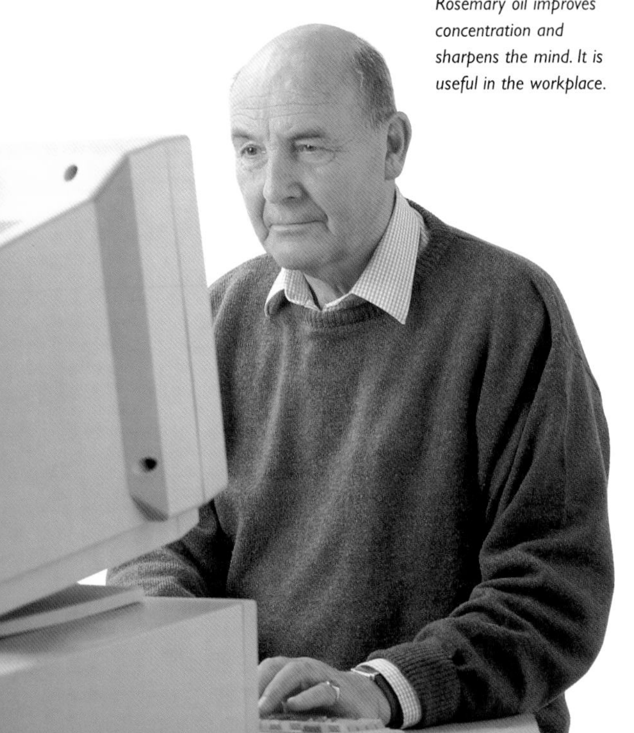

Rosemary oil improves concentration and sharpens the mind. It is useful in the workplace.

Fragrance profile: strong, camphoraceous, fresh, and herbal aroma with a definite eucalyptus tone.

Main uses: eases muscular aches and pains, backache, poor circulation; stimulates the scalp and eases dandruff; clears the breathing in colds, influenza, or sinusitis; stimulates the mind and wakes up the brain.

Suggested blends: for aches and pains and for poor circulation, try using 4 drops rosemary, 2 drops lemongrass, and 4 drops nutmeg in 4 teaspoons (20 ml) carrier oil.

For a hair and scalp tonic, try adding 5 drops rosemary and 5 drops tea tree to 4 teaspoons (20 ml) of unfragranced shampoo and then washing your hair as normal.

For easier breathing when suffering from colds or influenza, add 3 drops rosemary and 3 drops tea tree to a bowl of nearly boiling water and inhale the vapor for 20 minutes. To help stimulate the mind, vaporize 3 drops rosemary and 3 drops peppermint.

Cypress

Cupressus sempervirens

Plant profile: tall, evergreen cypress trees are an elegant feature of the landscape in Italy, France, Corsica, Sardinia, Spain, and Portugal. The Latin name *sempervirens* means "ever living," a reference to the long life of the species. They are often planted near dwellings or near churches to signify eternal life. The oil comes from the young twigs and leaves, which are highly aromatic. Distillation takes place mostly in France or Spain.

Safety information: no issues.

Fragrance profile: earthy, smoky, and green with camphoraceous and sweet notes.

Main uses: clears oily skin and blocked pores; improves lymphatic drainage and cellulite; eases spasmodic coughs and bronchitis; soothes fraught emotions.

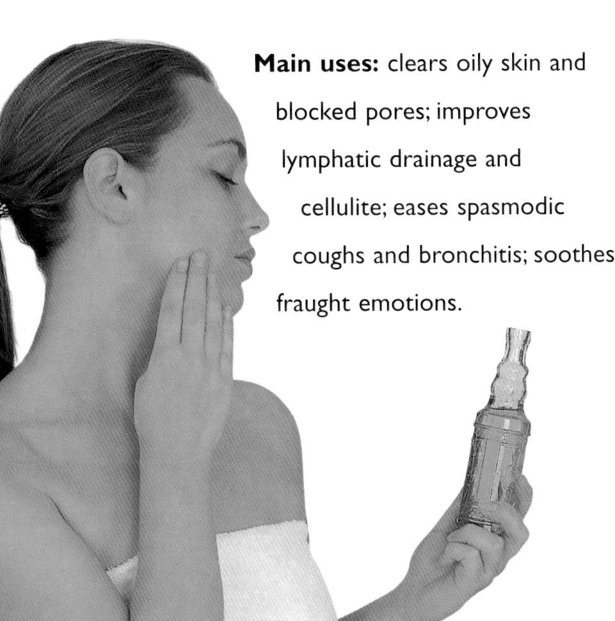

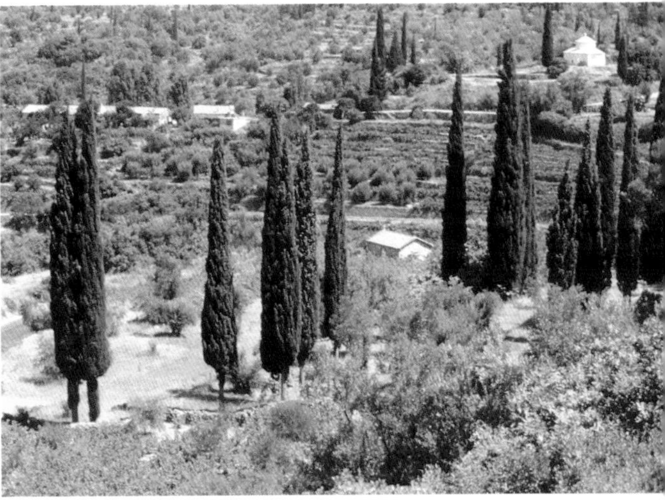

The tall dark shapes of cypress trees stand out clearly in a Mediterranean landscape.

Suggested blends: oily skin can be treated daily using 3 drops cypress, 3 drops tea tree, and 4 drops grapefruit in 4 teaspoons (20 ml) jojoba oil to cleanse and soothe the skin.

To counter cellulite, try using 4 drops cypress, 4 drops grapefruit, and 2 drops juniper in 4 teaspoons (20 ml) carrier oil for a vigorous daily massage of the affected areas.

To ease spasmodic coughs, do an inhalation with 3 drops cypress and 2 drops cedarwood twice daily; these oils can also be added to 2 teaspoons (10 ml) carrier oil and massaged into the chest.

If your emotions are overstretched or you are stressed, take a soothing bath with 3 drops cypress and 3 drops lavender and relax deeply.

Cypress essential oil is useful as a soothing skin treatment for an oily or blemished complexion.

Petitgrain (orange leaf)

Citrus aurantium* var. *amara

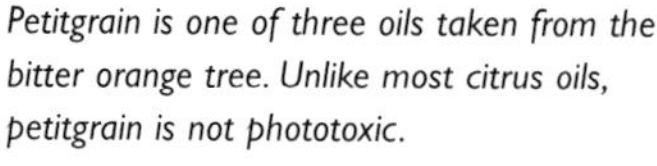

Petitgrain is one of three oils taken from the bitter orange tree. Unlike most citrus oils, petitgrain is not phototoxic.

Plant profile: petitgrain is one of three essential oils produced by the bitter orange tree. The leaves of the orange tree contain tiny sacs of essential oil, which are visible (like grains) to the naked eye when a leaf is held up to the sun—the French name of the oil means "little grain." The oil is an original ingredient of eau de cologne, popular since the eighteenth century. Most petitgrain oil comes from France or Paraguay.

Safety information: no issues. (Unlike orange, this oil is not phototoxic.)

Fragrance profile: a green, fresh, bittersweet aroma with a hint of citrus.

Main uses: tones, refreshes, and balances oily and combination skins; eases stomach cramps, indigestion, and wind; calms and soothes the mind, releasing tension and nervous exhaustion.

Suggested blends: for oily/combination skin, add 4 drops petitgrain, 2 drops patchouli, and 4 drops lavender to 4 teaspoons (20 ml) jojoba oil and use as a cleanser and skin-soother twice a day.

To ease stomach cramps, add 4 drops petitgrain, 2 drops peppermint, and 4 drops roman camomile to 4 teaspoons (20 ml) carrier oil and massage the abdomen (half the dose of drops in 4 teaspoons (20 ml) carrier can be used on children).

To relieve stress and calm the nerves, add 3 drops petitgrain and 3 drops sandalwood to a warm bath and relax.

Petitgrain is a fragrance note that can be found in many old-fashioned colognes.

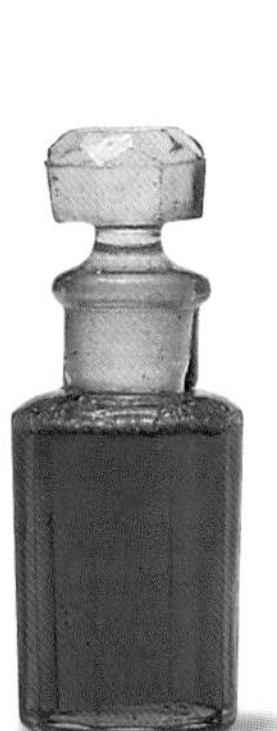
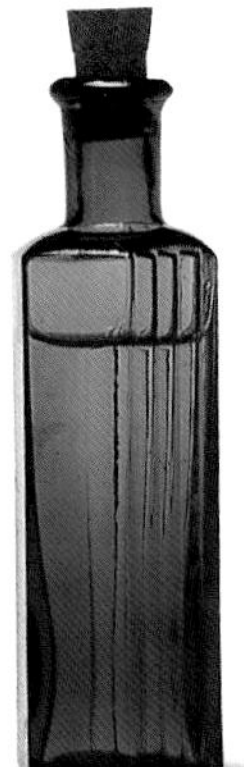
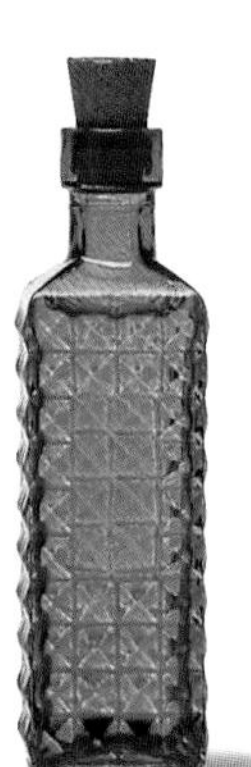
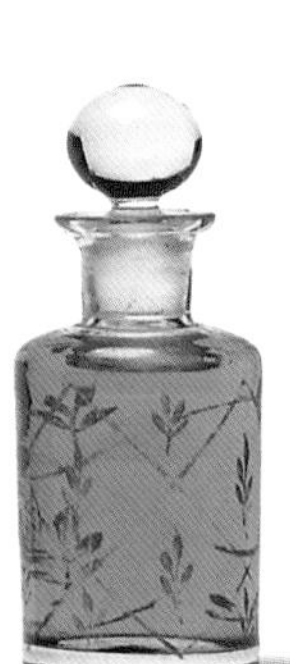
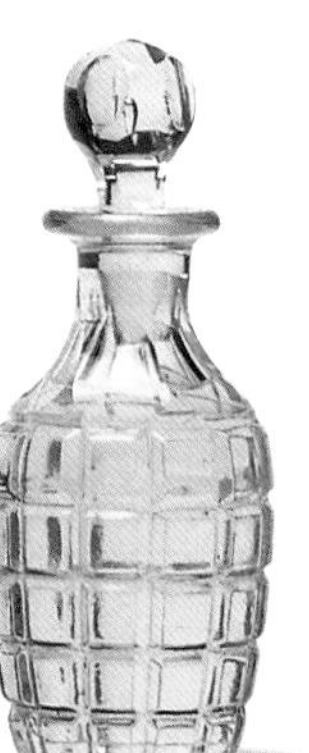
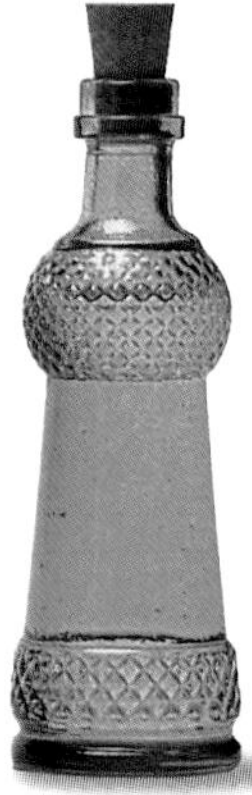

Patchouli

Pogostemon patchouli

Patchouli leaves are soft, velvety, and highly aromatic. The leaves are used in India to protect textiles from moths.

Plant profile: patchouli comes from India in the form of a thick, golden-brown essential oil with a very pronounced aroma. The leaves of the patchouli plant have a velvety texture thanks to thousands of tiny hairs on the surface. These contain microscopic sacs of essential oil, so that when you rub the leaf, the aroma is very strong on your fingers. Patchouli leaves are used to protect cloth from moths in India, and the oil is regarded as an insect repellent. It is also traditionally used in India as a skin conditioner and antiseptic.

Safety information: no issues.

Fragrance profile: a rich, velvety, musky aroma that develops spicy, earthy, and sweet tones with time.

Main uses: helps to soothe cracked, chapped, and dry skin and eczema; improves the complexion of mature and dry skins; increases sexual energy and helps to enhance sensuality.

Suggested blends: for dry, damaged, or cracked skin, try creating a massage blend of 3 drops patchouli, 3 drops cedarwood, and 4 drops roman camomile in 4 teaspoons (20 ml) jojoba oil and apply as needed.

To improve the complexion, add 3 drops patchouli, 4 drops frankincense, and 3 drops sandalwood to 4 teaspoons (20 ml) carrier oil and massage into the face, especially at night (this is appropriate for both men and women).

For a sensual massage blend, add 3 drops patchouli, 2 drops rose, and 5 drops orange to 4 teaspoons (20 ml) carrier oil.

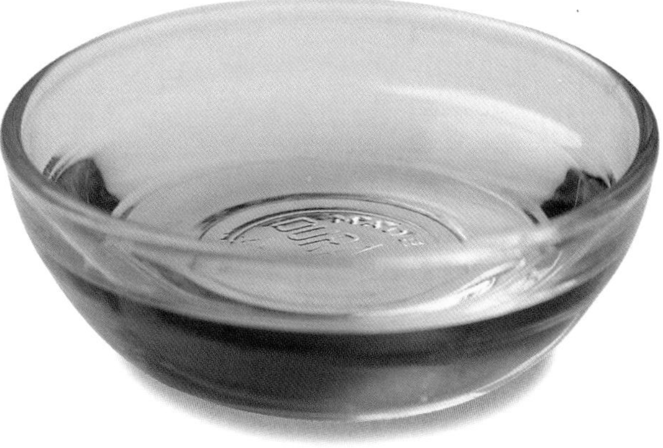

Patchouli makes a wonderful relaxing and sensual blend. The essential oil can increase and enhance sexual energy.

Eucalyptus

Eucalyptus globulus

Plant profile: there are more than 700 species of eucalyptus. In aromatherapy, several eucalyptus oils are used, of which *Eucalyptus globulus* is the most common. This evergreen tree from Australia can grow to a height of up to 300 feet (90 meters) when mature. The aromatic leaves are bluish-green on the upper surface and paler underneath. The leaves and the essential oil have been widely used as a household remedy in Australia from the days of the Aborigines to treat fevers, respiratory conditions, and skin infections.

Safety information: must not be swallowed—cases of severe internal poisoning have occurred. Safe on the skin or as an inhalation.

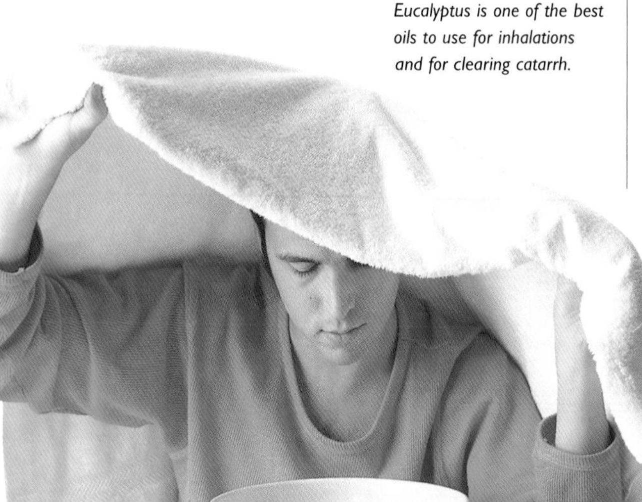

Eucalyptus is one of the best oils to use for inhalations and for clearing catarrh.

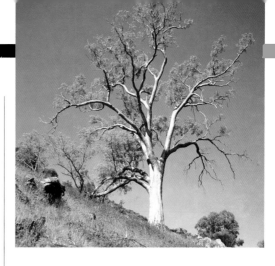

The eucalyptus tree is native to Australia and is an attractive evergreen with blue-green foliage.

Fragrance profile: extremely fresh and bracing, with woodier tones later.

Main uses: clears colds, blocked noses, sinusitis, chest infections; soothes burns, cuts, wounds, and insect bites; eases muscular pains; improves circulation; improves concentration.

Suggested blends: for colds and chest problems, use 2 drops eucalyptus and 3 drops tea tree in an inhalation twice daily. Add this combination of oils to 2 teaspoons (10 ml) carrier oil and massage into the chest area.

Use 4 teaspoons (20 ml) carrier oil. For damaged skin, add 2 drops eucalyptus, 3 drops tea tree, and 5 drops lavender, then apply twice daily.

For muscle pains, add 3 drops eucalyptus, 4 drops rosemary, and 3 drops ginger, and use for massage.

To improve concentration, vaporize 3 drops eucalyptus and 3 drops rosemary.

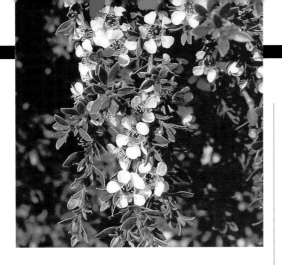

Tea tree essential oil is taken from the leaves of the tree and is very pungent and antiseptic.

Tea Tree

Melaleuca alternifolia

Plant profile: tea tree is native to Australia, where it has long been used by the aboriginal people as an antiseptic. The name "tea tree" refers to the practice of drinking an infusion of the leaves as a healing herbal drink, first observed by the sailors on Captain Cook's ship in the eighteenth century. Production of the oil is now a huge commercial enterprise with a whole host of tea tree products available on the market, from toothpaste to foot powder. It is one of the most antiseptic plants ever discovered.

Tea tree can help to treat the symptoms of influenza. Inhale the oil from a tissue whenever necessary.

Safety information: safe to use neat on the skin (2 drops on an absorbent cotton pad applied directly to the affected area) except on individuals with sensitive or allergy-prone skin, for whom it must be diluted in carrier oil.

Fragrance profile: medicinal, green, camphoraceous aroma, pungent and strong.

Main uses: clears skin infections and acne; heals wounds and cuts; soothes insect bites; clears athlete's foot; helps influenza, colds, bronchitis; boosts general immunity.

Suggested blends: for skin infections, add 4 drops tea tree, 3 drops sandalwood, and 3 drops lavender to 4 teaspoons (20 ml) carrier oil and apply as necessary. For chest problems, use an inhalation of 3 drops tea tree and 3 drops lemon twice daily. To boost immunity, add 2 drops tea tree, 2 drops bergamot, and 1 drop black pepper to a warm bath. Add these same oils to 2 teaspoons (10 ml) carrier oil and massage the upper chest area daily during an episode of influenza.

Lemongrass

Cymbopogon citratus

Plant profile: lemongrass is an aromatic tropical grass from India. It is well known as a flavoring ingredient in Indian and Thai cooking. In India, the grass is used in traditional medicine to help reduce fevers and kill infections, and also as an insect repellent. The leaves are chopped just above ground level and, as with all grasses, new shoots are then produced very quickly.

Safety information: the oil is regarded as a potential irritant to already sensitive or allergic skin and is not advised for infants and young children. It should always be diluted in a carrier, even in bath blends.

Fragrance profile: a very strong, "lemon sherbet" aroma that is zesty and sweet with a slightly heavy undertone.

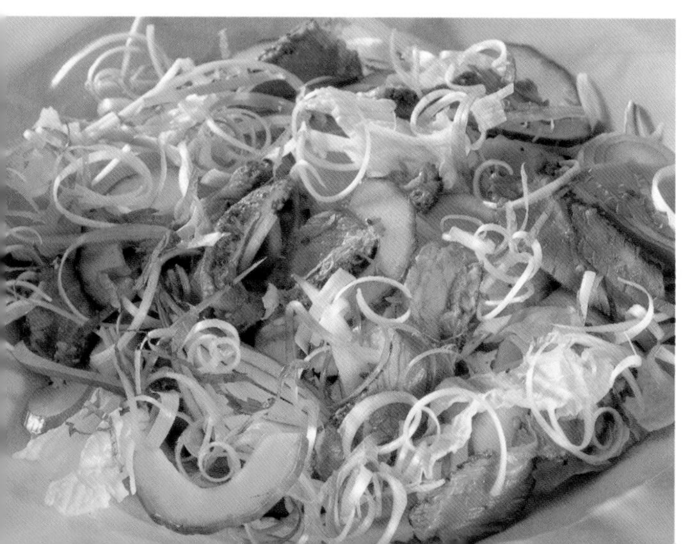

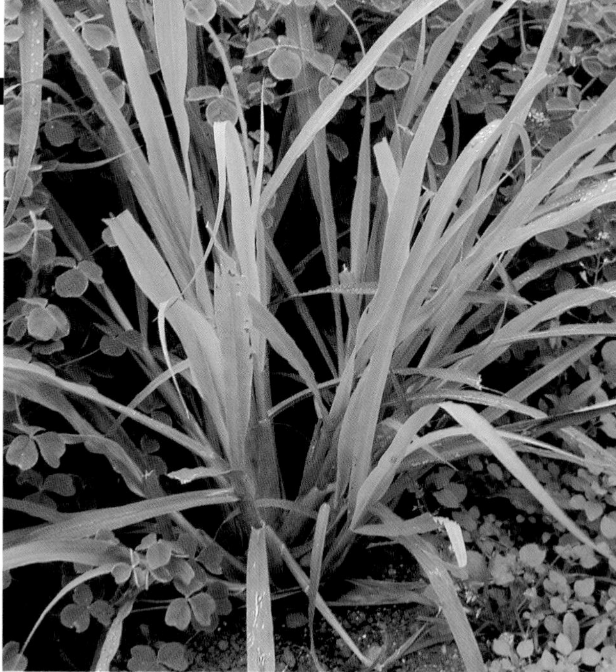

Lemongrass is a vigorous and aromatic tropical plant. It should always be diluted—even in blends for the bath.

Main uses: eases muscular aches, pains, and stiffness; eases stomach cramps, indigestion, and constipation; lifts depression or anxiety and improves the mood.

Suggested blends: for muscular aches, add 2 drops lemongrass, 3 drops rosemary, and 5 drops cardamom to 4 teaspoons (20 ml) carrier oil to massage the specific areas.

For stomach cramps or constipation, add 2 drops lemongrass, 4 drops coriander, and 4 drops nutmeg to 4 teaspoons (20 ml) carrier oil and massage the abdomen twice daily.

To improve mood and combat stress, add 2 drops lemongrass, 2 drops rose, and 6 drops frankincense to 4 teaspoons (20 ml) carrier oil.

Lemongrass is a key flavoring in most Thai dishes. Its zesty character can really lift a dish.

Palmarosa

Cymbopogon martini

Aromatic palmarosa is another grass grown in India. It has a similar fragrance to rose oil.

Plant profile: palmarosa is another aromatic grass from India, this time with a sweet smell and an altogether milder effect when used. In the past, it has often been used to adulterate or dilute pure rose oil, because the fragrance is somewhat similar and the grass is produced much more cheaply and in far larger quantities than rose. Palmarosa has a long-lasting aroma, which makes it a popular cosmetic ingredient in soaps, toiletries, and perfumes.

Safety information: no issues.

Fragrance profile: a long-lasting, sweet, and roselike aroma, which is soft and gentle with slightly lemony tones.

Main uses: soothes and calms irritated skin, acne, eczema, dermatitis; improves the facial complexion in all skin types, especially combination and mature; soothes cystitis and clears urinary tract infections; calms and de-stresses the nerves.

Suggested blends: Use 4 teaspoons (20 ml) carrier oil. For sensitive or irritated skin, add 3 drops palmarosa and 2 drops roman camomile (note the low dilution) and apply as needed.

To balance and rejuvenate the complexion, add 4 drops palmarosa, 3 drops frankincense, and 3 drops sandalwood and massage the face, especially at night. To uplift your mood, add 3 drops palmarosa, 4 drops grapefruit, and 3 drops orange, for an exotic and soft massage blend. For cystitis or urinary problems, add 3 drops palmarosa and 3 drops sandalwood to a warm bath to soothe the area.

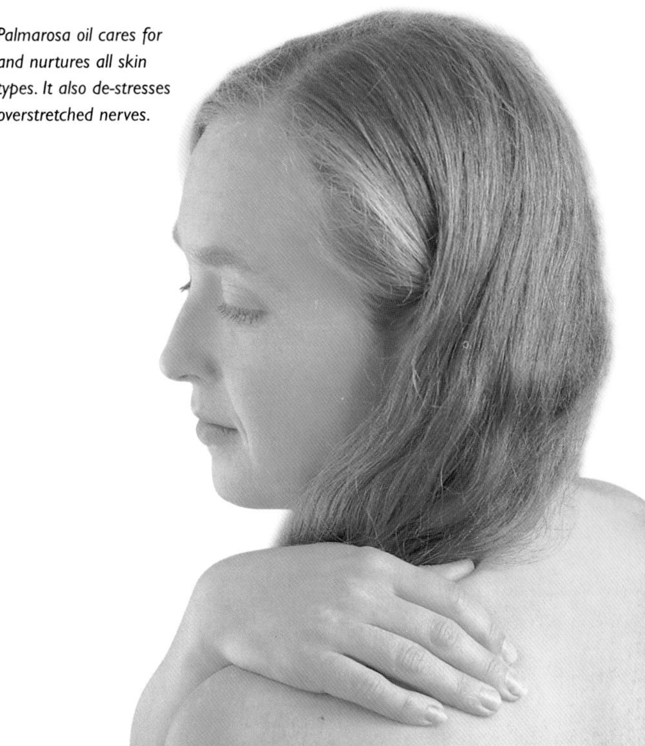

Palmarosa oil cares for and nurtures all skin types. It also de-stresses overstretched nerves.

Flower Oils

These are some of the most exquisite fragrances you will encounter. Captured from the petals, they are the unique aromatic signal of that plant.

Lavender

Lavandula angustifolia

Plant profile: lavender oil is now widely produced in the UK, southern France, Tasmania, New Zealand, and Bulgaria. Purple lavender fields make one of the most wonderful aromatic landscapes, filled with bees and butterflies busily enjoying the magnificent supply of pollen. Lavender oils vary in fragrance according to the altitude where they are produced—high altitude oils have sharper and fresher aromas, and low altitude ones are sweeter and softer.

Safety information: no issues. Lavender can be used neat (2 drops on an absorbent cotton pad applied directly to the affected area).

Fragrance profile: mainly soft, sweet, and floral with camphoraceous and pungent notes.

Main uses: soothes cuts, burns, wounds, insect bites, sore skin; eases headaches, migraine, and muscular aches and tension; soothes chesty spasmodic coughs; helps insomnia, nervous tension, and anxiety; useful for both adults and children.

Suggested blends: for skin problems, add 4 drops lavender, 3 drops tea tree, and 3 drops roman camomile to 4 teaspoons (20 ml) carrier oil and massage into the affected area.

Ease headaches by adding 3 drops lavender to 1 teaspoon (5 ml) carrier oil and massaging the forehead and neck to provide relief.

To relieve coughs, an inhalation with 4 drops lavender and 3 drops cedarwood done twice daily can often be helpful.

To ease insomnia, vaporize 3 drops lavender and 3 drops orange to help you fall asleep.

Lavender fields are vibrantly purple and wonderfully aromatic. Bees and butterflies love visiting the plants that grow here.

Geranium

Pelargonium graveolens

Plant profile: this is a tropical geranium with velvety, frilly leaves. Rubbing the tiny surface hairs releases a strong, rosy aroma onto your fingers. The geranium grows as a shrub up to 3 feet (1 meter) in height and has pinkish flowers. The essential oil has a powerful floral aroma. The island of Réunion in the Indian Ocean produces the best-quality oil. Chinese and Egyptian geranium oils are also available but have a much heavier fragrance.

The leaves of this geranium release a strong rosy aroma.

Safety information: no issues.

Fragrance profile: rosy, sweet, and strong, with a hint of lemon and fresh green notes.

Main uses: soothes cracked and inflamed skin, eczema, dermatitis, acne, and congested or oily skin; eases premenstrual symptoms such as lack of energy, bloatedness, and fluid retention; soothes mood swings and helps to balance hormonally related emotional upsets.

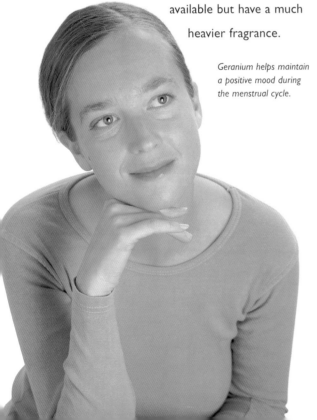

Geranium helps maintain a positive mood during the menstrual cycle.

Suggested blends: for skin problems, add 3 drops geranium, 3 drops sandalwood, and 4 drops lavender to 4 teaspoons (20 ml) carrier oil and apply to the area as needed.

To ease premenstrual symptoms, try adding 2 drops geranium and 3 drops petitgrain to a warm bath. You can also use the same combination of oils in 2 teaspoons (10 ml) carrier oil for an uplifting massage afterward.

To help balance mood swings, add 3 drops geranium, 3 drops lemon, and 4 drops orange to 4 teaspoons (20 ml) carrier oil and massage into your skin for a floral and citrus uplift.

Ylang Ylang

Cananga odorata

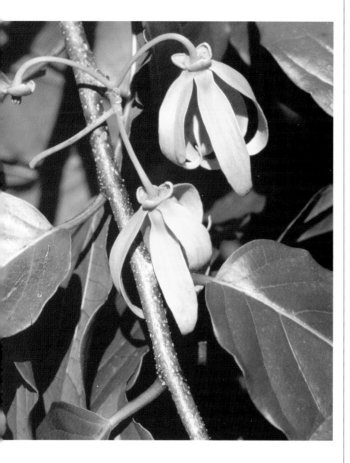

Ylang ylang flowers are beautiful exotic blooms, which yield large amounts of deeply scented essential oil.

Plant profile: from Madagascar, an island off the coast of East Africa, comes the "flower of flowers"—ylang ylang. Beautiful, lush, golden-yellow flowers with velvety petals produce a wonderful oil very similar to jasmine. There is such a high content of fragrance in the flowers that the essential oil can be drawn off three times during the process of distillation, offering three grades of essential oil. The first collection of oil is known as the "perfume" grade and is the best quality.

Safety information: no major issues. Some individuals find the strong floral aroma brings on a headache.

Fragrance profile: sharp and sweet, becoming deeply floral, jasmine-like, heady, and soft with time.

Main uses: tones oily and combination skins; reduces panic attacks and stress-related anxiety symptoms; soothes and calms emotional stress and overstretched nerves.

Suggested blends: to tone oily skin, add 2 drops ylang ylang, 3 drops sandalwood, and 5 drops frankincense to 4 teaspoons (20 ml) jojoba oil and use as a cleanser and skin-soother twice daily.

For panic and anxiety attacks, add 2 drops ylang ylang and 3 drops lavender to a warm bath, and add the same combination of oils to 2 teaspoons (10 ml) carrier oil for a relaxing neck and shoulder massage afterward.

To soothe the nerves and ease anxiety, add 2 drops ylang ylang, 2 drops patchouli, and 5 drops orange to 4 teaspoons (20 ml) carrier oil and massage your body gently.

Rose

Rosa damascena

Plant profile: costly and labor-intensive to produce, rose is one of the most beautiful of all essential oils. The little damask rose from Kazanlik in Bulgaria produces the finest quality rose oil, although Turkish, Moroccan, and Russian rose oils are also excellent. Rose "otto" is simply distilled rose oil—between 50 and 100 blooms are needed per drop. An "absolute" of rose, chemically extracted, is also available at a lower cost. Look out for pure rose oil already diluted in jojoba as a more affordable and still effective way to use this oil.

Safety information: no issues.

Fragrance profile: honey-sweet, slightly lemony, and soft, with richness and depth.

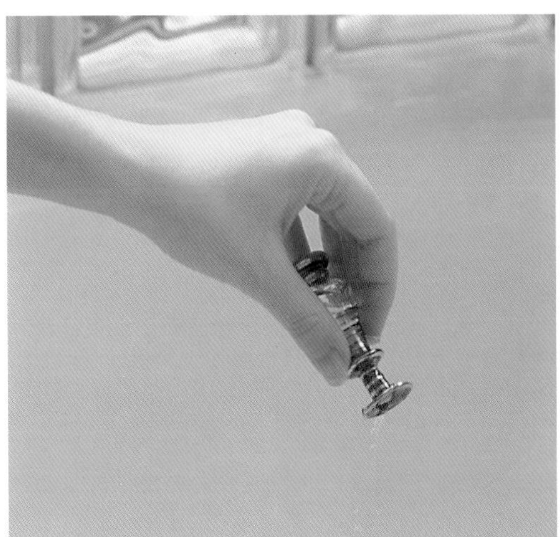

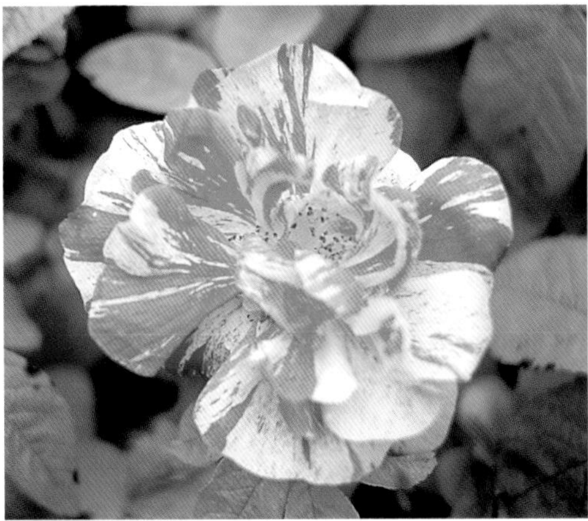

The damask rose has a uniquely glorious aroma. It is one of the most costly oils to produce but is worth every drop.

Main uses: tones and rejuvenates all skin types, especially dry, sensitive, and mature; eases premenstrual and menopausal symptoms; helps release feelings of grief and separation, restoring the heart.

Suggested blends: to tone the skin, add 2 drops rose, 4 drops frankincense, and 4 drops sandalwood to 4 teaspoons (20 ml) jojoba oil (halve the number of drops for sensitive skin). For premenstrual or menopausal symptoms, add 4 drops rose, 3 drops neroli, and 3 drops mandarin to 4 teaspoons (20 ml) carrier oil and massage into the body. To ease grief, add 2 drops rose and 3 drops orange to a bath. Use the same combination in 2 teaspoons (10 ml) carrier oil for a massage afterward.

Pure rose oil trickled into a bath releases an amazing fragrance, which can relieve stress almost instantly.

Roman Camomile

Anthemis nobilis

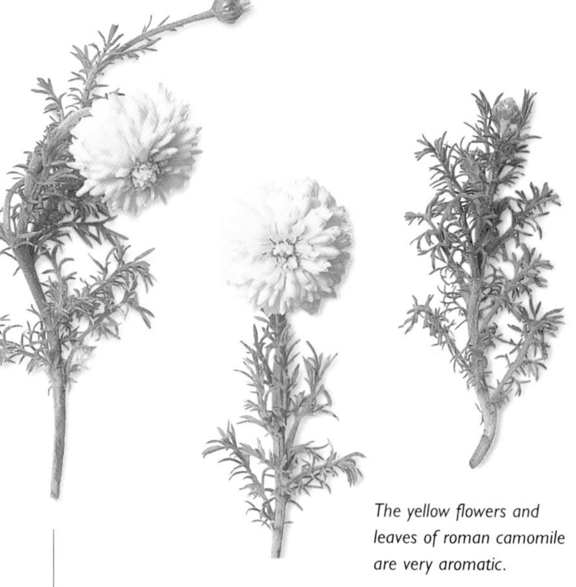

The yellow flowers and leaves of roman camomile are very aromatic.

Plant profile: the name "camomile" is originally from the Greek *kamaimelon,* meaning "ground apple." This derives from the fact that the plant is low-growing and smells strongly of apples. In its non-flowering variety, this species of camomile is often used to make a fragrant lawn. The flowers, however, are required for distillation.

The oil has a pale blue color due to the presence of a substance called "azulene," which has anti-inflammatory properties. The oil is now cultivated successfully in the UK.

Safety information: no issues.

Fragrance profile: fruity (apple-like), sweet, fresh, and soft.

Main uses: soothes cuts, burns, sore, dry skin, nappy rash; eases menstrual cramps, premenstrual low energy, and tension; soothes headaches, migraine; helps insomnia, nervous exhaustion, tension, restlessness, and stress-related problems.

Suggested blends: Use 4 teaspoons (20 ml) carrier oil. For skin problems, add 3 drops roman camomile, 4 drops lavender, and 3 drops palmarosa and apply as necessary; for baby nappy rash, use 1 drop only of camomile for an extremely gentle application.

For menstrual symptoms, add 3 drops roman camomile and 2 drops marjoram to a warm bath, then add this blend of oils to 2 teaspoons (10 ml) carrier oil and massage the lower abdomen.

For insomnia and restlessness, try vaporizing 3 drops roman camomile and 3 drops lavender in the bedroom before turning in for the night.

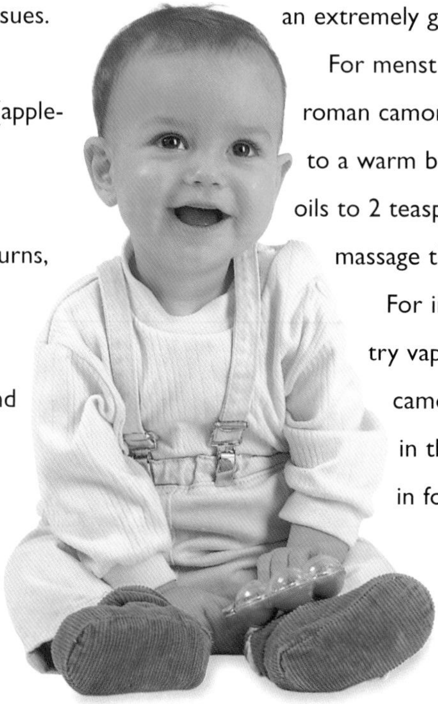

Babies and younger children respond well to the fragrance of roman camomile essential oil.

Neroli (orange blossom)

Citrus aurantium* var. *amara

Plant profile: the essential oil from orange blossom is named after princess Neroli, an Italian noblewoman of the Renaissance period who perfumed her gloves with Neroli flowers. The oil has an enchanting aroma, and is costly and labor-intensive to produce, as the fragrant white flowers of the bitter orange tree have to be picked by hand. Neroli essential oil is mostly distilled in France and Morocco. Look out for pure neroli diluted in jojoba from quality essential oil ranges, as this is a more affordable way of trying this fragrance.

Safety information: no issues.

Fragrance profile: creamy-sweet, citrusy, rich, and soft with green undertones.

Main uses: tones and rejuvenates the complexion, especially dry, mature, or undernourished skins; helps scar tissue, wounds, and cuts; eases nervous indigestion and irritable bowel symptoms; helps calm panic, shock, and sudden emotional upsets.

Suggested blends: for skincare, add 3 drops neroli, 4 drops frankincense, and 3 drops patchouli to 4 teaspoons (20 ml) jojoba for a nourishing facial massage oil.

To heal damaged skin, add 3 drops neroli, 4 drops lavender, and 4 drops myrrh to 4 teaspoons (20 ml) carrier oil and apply to the area twice daily. For nervous indigestion, add 4 drops neroli, 3 drops peppermint, and 3 drops ginger to 4 teaspoons (20 ml) carrier oil for gentle abdominal massage as necessary.

To help shock and panic, simply place 2 drops neroli on a tissue and inhale the fragrance until calm is restored.

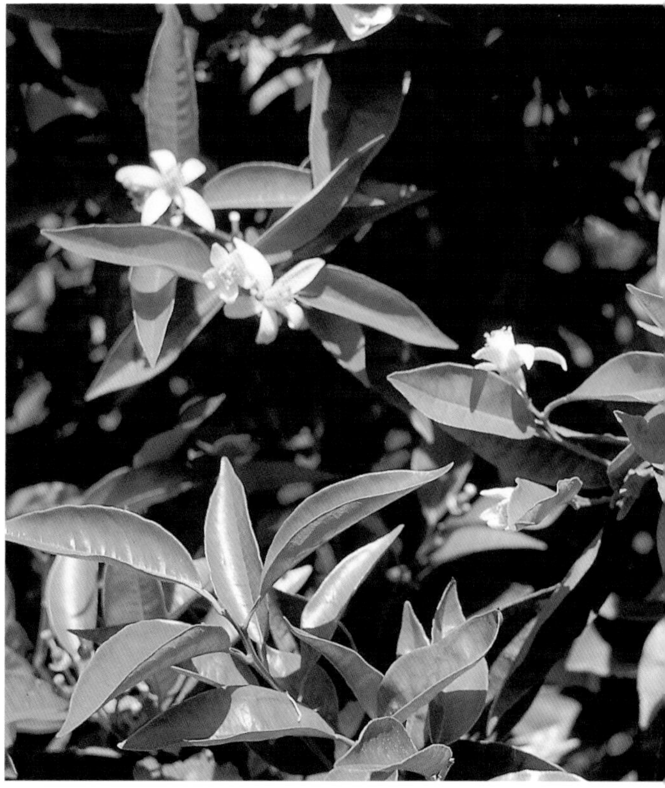

Each orange blossom has to be picked by hand, making neroli—along with rose—one of the more expensive essential oils.

Berry and Seed Oils

These are aromatic packages of pungent fragrance, often designed to attract animals and birds. They ingest the seeds and then eventually release them into the earth, helping plant reproduction.

Nutmeg

Myristica fragrans

Aromatic nutmegs have a spicy, cheering fragrance. They can be used in cakes and biscuits to give a distinctive flavor.

Plant profile: the nutmeg tree grows in Indonesia and Sri Lanka. The fruits are covered with a layer called mace, which is removed before processing. The highly aromatic nutmegs are steam-distilled to give a fragrant essential oil. In Western herbal tradition, nutmegs were prized for their digestive tonic and muscle-warming properties. In medieval times they were so valuable they were kept locked away.

Safety information: a strong oil, so should be used in moderation.

Fragrance profile: warm, sharp, spicy, and sweet with a distinctive softness later.

Main uses: eases muscular aches and pains, arthritic pain, and cold extremities; soothes and calms indigestion, stomach cramps, nausea; helps to re-energize the body after illness, speeding convalescence, uplifting the spirits, and restoring the circulation.

Suggested blends: Use 4 teaspoons (20 ml) carrier oil. For aches and pains, add 2 drops nutmeg, 4 drops cardamom, and 4 drops grapefruit, and massage into the affected area. To soothe the digestion, add 2 drops nutmeg, 4 drops peppermint, and 4 drops ginger for an abdominal massage. As a restoring tonic, add 1 drop nutmeg, 2 drops black pepper, and 2 drops orange to a warm bath and relax in the water. Add the same oils to 2 teaspoons (10 ml) carrier oil and massage into the skin afterward.

Blends made using nutmeg can ease muscular cramps.

Black Pepper

Piper nigrum

Plant profile: this plant is a trailing vinelike climber with lovely, heart-shaped, dark green leaves and clusters of white flowers that become the berries—or peppercorns. These turn from red to black as they mature (white pepper has had the outer layer removed). Black peppercorns are steam-distilled to yield the essential oil. The tropical plant is native to India, and the oil is produced there as well as in Indonesia and Malaysia.

Safety information: no issues.

Fragrance profile: warm, musty, sharp, and spicy, with heavier sweet notes later.

Main uses: warms and stimulates blood circulation; helps to ease aches and pains; soothes indigestion, stomach cramps, and constipation; strengthens the immune system, especially against influenza.

Suggested blends: to help stimulate poor or sluggish circulation, add 4 drops black pepper, 2 drops lemongrass, and 4 drops cardamom to 4 teaspoons (20 ml) carrier oil and massage into the affected area as needed.

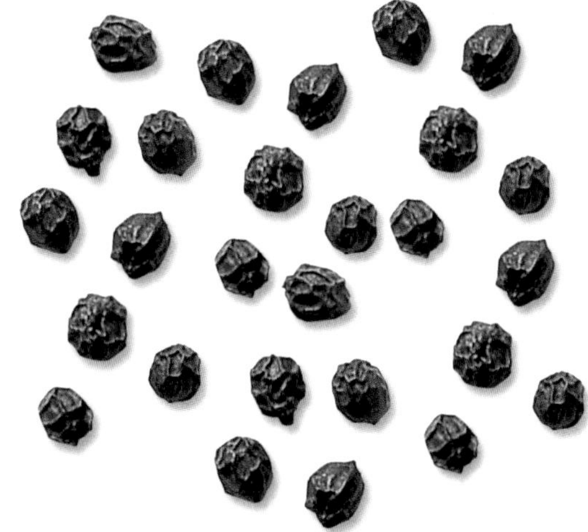

Black peppercorns yield a warm and pungent oil, which has a very spicy aroma. Black pepper essential oil can boost the immune system and ease indigestion.

To ease indigestion or constipation, add 3 drops black pepper, 3 drops peppermint, and 4 drops neroli to 4 teaspoons (20 ml) carrier oil and massage the abdomen twice daily.

To boost the immune system, add 1 drop black pepper, 2 drops tea tree, and 2 drops bergamot to an evening bath and soak for at least 20 minutes. Add these oils to 4 teaspoons (20 ml) carrier oil and massage the chest area afterward.

Poor circulation can be helped by vigorously massaging the area in question with the pepper blend.

Cardamom

Elettaria cardamomum

Essential oils like cardamom improve the mood and warm the affected areas. Cardamom is a good energy tonic too.

Plant profile: a member of the same plant family as ginger, cardamom produces aromatic flowers that turn into little seed pods filled with tiny black seeds. The pods are traditionally chewed in India to sweeten the breath after eating spicy food, and the wonderful aroma of cardamom is also used to flavor Indian ice cream and confectionery. Cardamom is commonly used in Eastern medicinal traditions as a lung tonic and immunity-boosting plant remedy.

Safety information: no issues.

Fragrance profile: warm, fruity, sweet, and spicy with a mouthwatering pungent freshness.

Main uses: soothes and opens the chest, helping breathing and congestion; warms and soothes stomach cramps and indigestion; uplifts the mind and gives a positive feeling when energy is low.

Suggested blends: to improve breathing, add 3 drops cardamom and 2 drops cedarwood to nearly boiling water and inhale the vapor, repeating twice daily; add the same oils to 2 teaspoons (10 ml) carrier oil and massage the chest area afterward.

To ease digestion problems, massage the abdomen twice daily with 3 drops cardamom, 3 drops coriander, and 4 drops orange in 4 teaspoons (20 ml) carrier oil.

As a tonic to raise low spirits, add 3 drops cardamom and 2 drops mandarin to a warm bath and relax in the water. Add the same oils to 2 teaspoons (10 ml) carrier oil and massage into the skin afterward.

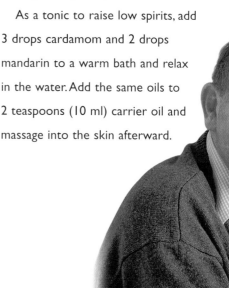

May Chang

Litsea cubeba

May chang has berries that smell like lemon sherbet! It is not a suitable oil for babies and young children.

Plant profile: a tree from China with delicate leaves and little whitish-yellow flowers that become highly lemon-scented tiny fruits. The oil from the berries of the may chang tree is used a great deal in China as a mood enhancer and as a tonic to the heart; it calms and regulates the heart rhythm when used in massage. It is similar to lemongrass, but has a much lighter and sweeter fragrance.

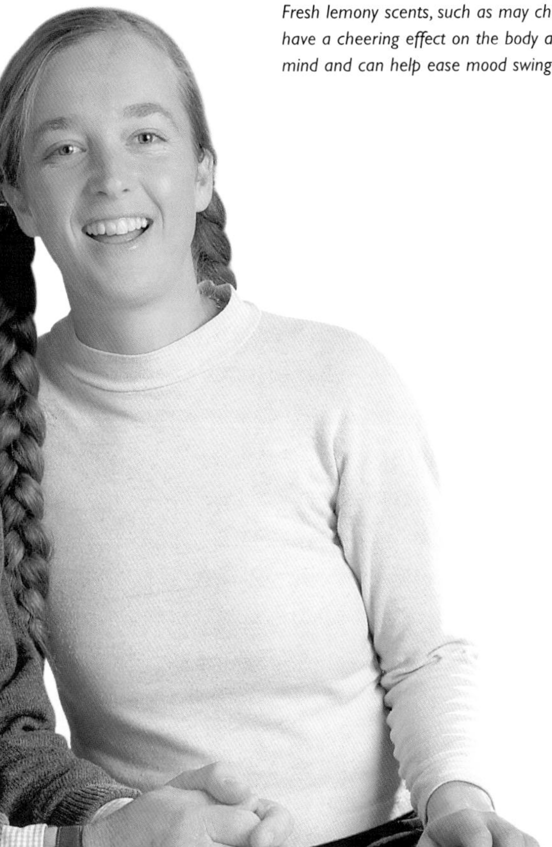

Fresh lemony scents, such as may chang, have a cheering effect on the body and mind and can help ease mood swings.

Safety information: avoid using this oil on sensitive or damaged skin. It is not suitable for babies or children. Always dilute this oil, even if you are using it in the bath.

Fragrance profile: soft, sweet, and fruity with a strong "lemon sherbet" aroma that is zesty and mouthwatering.

Main uses: eases muscular aches and pains, strains, and backache; eases panic or stress attacks; uplifts depression and anxiety, mood swings, and tearfulness.

Suggested blends: for aches and pains, add 2 drops may chang, 4 drops juniper, and 4 drops lavender and massage affected areas.

Panic and stress attacks can be eased by simply placing 2 drops may chang on a tissue and inhaling the aroma for a few minutes. Add 2 drops may chang and 3 drops neroli to a warm bath and relax in the water to recover.

Uplift moods and ease depression by a massage with a blend of 2 drops may chang, 2 drops rose, and 6 drops frankincense in 4 teaspoons (20 ml) carrier oil.

Juniper

Juniperus communis

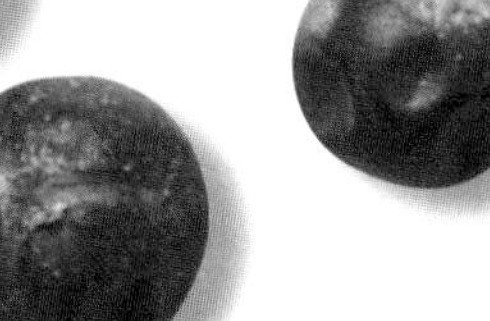

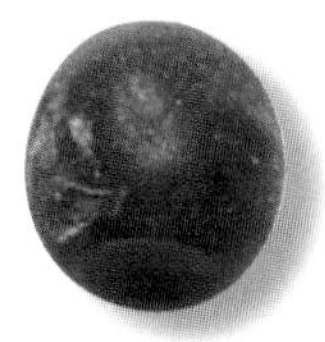

Blue-black juniper berries are sharp and pungently scented. They take up to two years to turn black.

Plant profile: juniper is a vigorous shrub with dark green spiky leaves. The essential oil comes mainly from Germany, where the plant grows well, and also from parts of Croatia. The berries on the juniper bush take up to two years to turn black and produce the best-quality oil. Juniper is also used in making gin, and in northern European cooking it is used to give pungent flavor to root vegetables. In herbal medicine, juniper is considered to be a strong diuretic and internal cleanser.

Safety information: this is best avoided during pregnancy, and also by people with any serious kidney complaints.

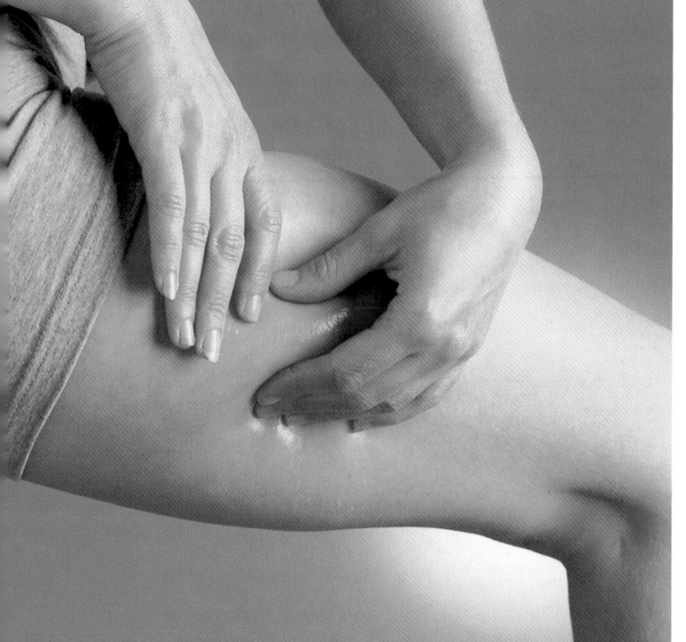

Fragrance profile: pungent, peppery, and camphoraceous, with sweeter, softer notes developing later.

Main uses: helps to clear lymphatic congestion and detoxify the system; opens the chest and eases breathing in respiratory complaints; freshens the mind and helps improve concentration.

Suggested blends: to help detoxify, add 2 drops juniper, 2 drops angelica, and 6 drops grapefruit to 4 teaspoons (20 ml) carrier oil for a vigorous daily massage to affected areas of the body.

To help respiratory complaints, add 2 drops juniper and 3 drops eucalyptus to a bowl of nearly boiling water and inhale the vapors. Do this twice daily. To help concentration, vaporize 3 drops juniper and 3 drops lemon in a room; this also helps to clear the atmosphere and neutralize any stale or unpleasant odors.

Massage blends with juniper can help improve areas of poor circulation in the legs. A vigorous daily massage is recommended.

Coriander Seed

Coriandrum sativum

Plant profile: the coriander plant is a highly aromatic herb with deliciously flavored dark green leaves (cilantro). It is easy to grow and makes a pungent addition to salad greens and a wonderful garnish for Indian dishes. The coriander plant produces umbels—umbrella-like stalks topped with little white flowers that eventually turn to brownish-colored aromatic seeds. These are distilled to produce the essential oil in Eastern European countries, including Russia and Croatia.

Safety information: no issues.

Fragrance profile: woody, spicy, and sweet with a slight hint of musk.

Main uses: warms and soothes muscular stiffness and aching joints; helps build immunity, especially in the case of influenza; eases mental exhaustion and overstretched nerves.

Coriander is a herb widely used in cooking and herbalism. It has attractive heads of white flowers.

Coriander seeds are a pungent spice and are used frequently in Indian cuisine. The leaves are also used as a delicious garnish.

Suggested blends: to warm muscles, add 3 drops coriander, 3 drops black pepper, and 4 drops ginger to 4 teaspoons (20 ml) carrier oil; massage twice daily. To boost the immune system, add 2 drops coriander and 3 drops lemon to a bath; then add the same oils to 2 teaspoons (10 ml) carrier oil and massage into the chest area. To ease exhaustion, add 2 drops coriander, 1 drop neroli, and 2 drops lavender to a bath; add the same oils to 2 teaspoons (10 ml) carrier oil afterward for a massage. This routine can also help improve sleep quality.

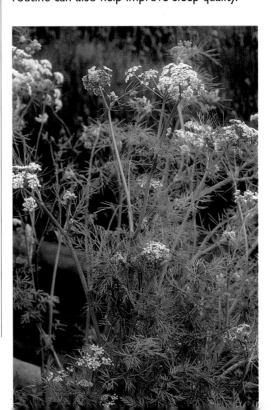

Fruit Oils

These oils are packed into tiny fragrant globules in the rind of citrus fruit. Fresh and zesty, they are mouthwatering aromas, loved by adults and children.

Orange (sweet)

Citrus sinensis

Plant profile: most orange essential oil that is commercially available is from the sweet orange tree, which originated in China. The essential oil is expressed, or crushed out of the rind of the fruit. The bitter orange tree (*Citrus aurantium*) produces petitgrain and neroli essential oils.

Safety information: very mildly phototoxic; avoid exposure to strong sunlight or a sunbed for 12 hours after skin application.

Fragrance profile: sweet, warm, fresh, and citrusy.

Main uses: soothes stomach cramps and indigestion (especially in children); rejuvenates congested and slack skin; uplifts depression, mood swings, anxiety, and emotional stress.

Children particularly love the sweet soft aroma of orange essential oil. It is a popular festive smell!

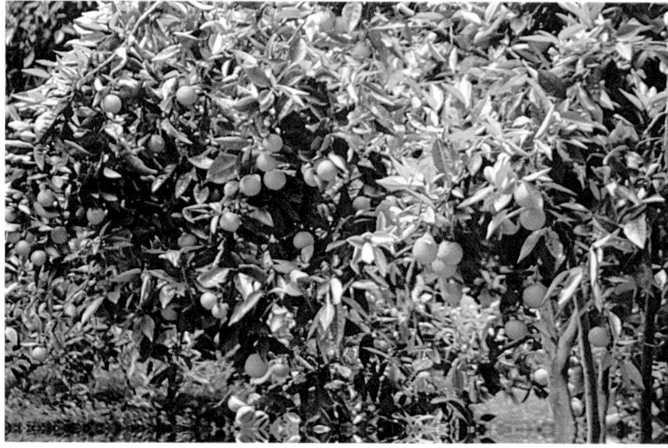

Orange trees are covered with delicious-smelling leaves, flowers, and fruits. Orange essential oil is popular with young and old alike.

Suggested blends: for stomach problems, add 4 drops orange, 2 drops peppermint, and 4 drops ginger to 4 teaspoons (20 ml) carrier oil and massage the abdomen 2–3 times daily (halve the number of drops for children).

To rejuvenate tired skin, add 4 drops orange, 4 drops frankincense, and 2 drops cypress to 4 teaspoons (20 ml) jojoba. For anxiety, add 2 drops orange, 1 drop rose, and 2 drops sandalwood to a bath; use this blend in 2 teaspoons (10 ml) carrier oil for massage.

Lemon

Citrus limonum

Lemon rind is packed full of fresh and zesty essential oil. It is a good oil to assist concentration and sharpen the mind.

Plant profile: the finest essential oil of lemon is considered to come from trees grown in Sicily, although the fruit is also cultivated in California, Florida, and Israel. The evergreen tree is thorny and has shiny, dark green, aromatic leaves that produce an essential oil called *petitgrain citronnier*. The fragrant flowers turn into the fruit, which when ripe are a warm golden yellow. Essential oil of lemon is expressed, or squeezed out of the peel of the fruit.

Safety information: mildly phototoxic; avoid any exposure to strong sunlight or a sunbed for at least 12 hours after application of the oil to the skin.

Fragrance profile: green, citrusy, and fresh, zesty, and bright; softer and more sherbety tones develop with time.

Main uses: helps build immunity against colds, influenza, and other viral infections; detoxifies the system and assists lymphatic drainage; freshens the mind and helps to improve concentration.

Lemon trees grow all over the Mediterranean, and particularly in Sicily. They are a wonderful sight in the summer.

Suggested blends: to help boost the immune system, vaporize 3 drops lemon and 2 drops tea tree to disinfect the air; add the same oils to 2 teaspoons (10 ml) carrier oil to massage the chest area twice daily.

To help detoxify the body, add 4 drops lemon, 2 drops angelica, and 4 drops juniper to 4 teaspoons (20 ml) carrier oil and massage the legs and other affected areas twice daily.

To assist concentration and improve alertness, add 3 drops lemon and 3 drops rosemary to a vaporizer; this is especially helpful when studying.

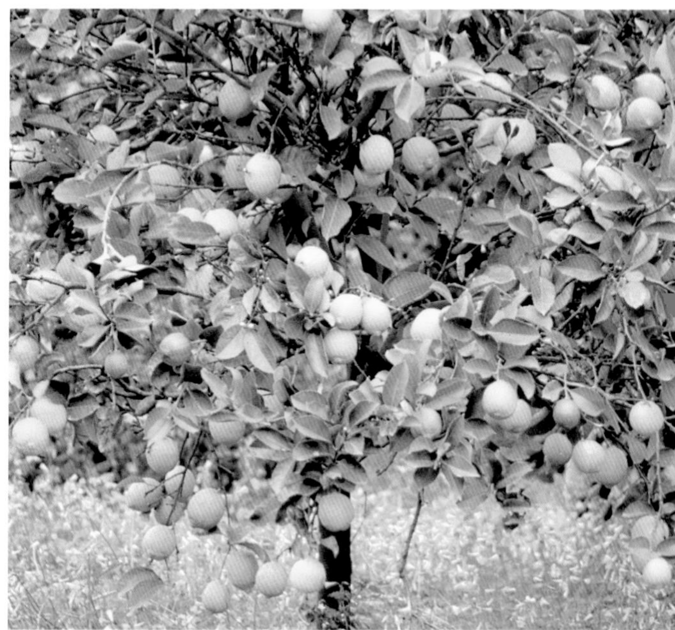

Mandarin

Citrus reticulata

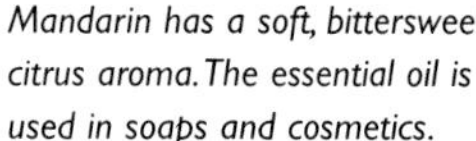

Mandarin has a soft, bittersweet citrus aroma. The essential oil is used in soaps and cosmetics.

Plant profile: this small citrus tree is evergreen and its fruit has an immediate association with festive celebrations. The fruit and the expressed oil are produced mainly in Brazil, Spain, and Italy. Because it is so mild and pleasant, mandarin is used as a flavoring in many confectionery items, liqueurs, and soft drinks, as well as in soaps, toiletries, and perfumes. It is a favorite with children.

Safety information: very mildly phototoxic; avoid exposure to strong sunlight or a sunbed for 12 hours after application to the skin.

Fragrance profile: fresh, pungent, and sweet with a bright citrus zest; softer and more floral tones developing with time.

Main uses: clears congested and oily skin; soothes stomach cramps and nervous indigestion (especially in children); eases insomnia, restless sleep, and troubled dreams.

Suggested blends: for oily skin, add 4 drops mandarin, 3 drops cypress, and 3 drops juniper to 4 teaspoons (20 ml) jojoba oil and use as a cleanser and skin-soother at night.

To ease digestion problems, add 4 drops mandarin, 4 drops lavender, and 2 drops roman camomile to 4 teaspoons (20 ml) carrier oil and gently massage the abdomen twice daily (halve the number of drops for children).

To help induce restful sleep, add 3 drops mandarin and 3 drops lavender to a vaporizer.

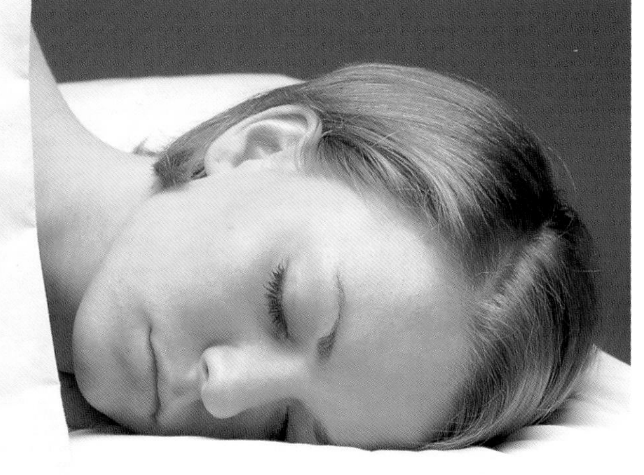

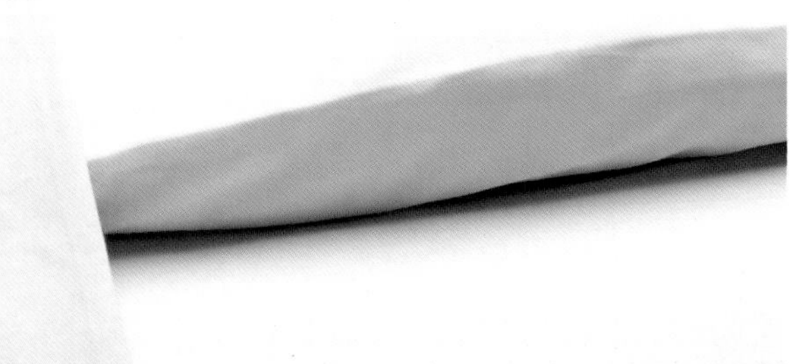

Vaporizing mandarin essential oil at night helps to improve sleep and ease any lingering anxiety.

Grapefruit

Citrus x paradisi

The large golden grapefruit produces a different aroma to its other citrus relatives.

Plant profile: grapefruit is a hybrid which may have been derived from an old variety of fruit called the shaddock. It is now cultivated extensively in Florida in its familiar golden and pink-fleshed varieties. The essential oil is expressed from the peel, and grapefruit has an aroma quite different from its citrus relatives, thanks to the presence of sharp bitter constituents that give it freshness and zest.

Safety information: mildly phototoxic; avoid exposure to strong sunlight or a sunbed for 12 hours after application to the skin.

Fragrance profile: green, bittersweet, zesty, and fresh, with a soft, powdery afternote.

Main uses: helps clear toxins and improve areas of cellulite; eases the chest and breathing in colds and influenza; eases anxiety, depression, and stress, helps to relieve insomnia and disturbed dreams.

Suggested blends: to detoxify, first use a skin brush on dry skin to boost the circulation, then add 4 drops grapefruit, 3 drops lemon, and 3 drops juniper to 4 teaspoons (20 ml) carrier oil for an evening massage of the affected areas.

To relieve chest infections, add 3 drops grapefruit and 2 drops cedarwood to a bowl of nearly boiling water and inhale the vapor for 20 minutes; add the same drops to 2 teaspoons (10 ml) carrier oil afterward and massage the chest.

To ease insomnia and anxiety, add 2 drops grapefruit and 3 drops sandalwood to a warm bath and relax in the water; add the same drops to 2 teaspoons (10 ml) carrier oil and massage the skin afterward.

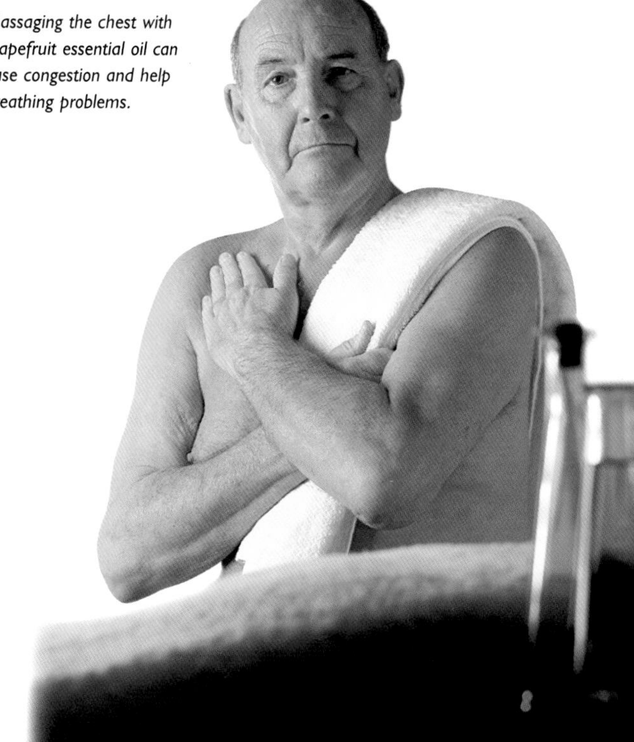

Massaging the chest with grapefruit essential oil can ease congestion and help breathing problems.

Bergamot

Citrus bergamia

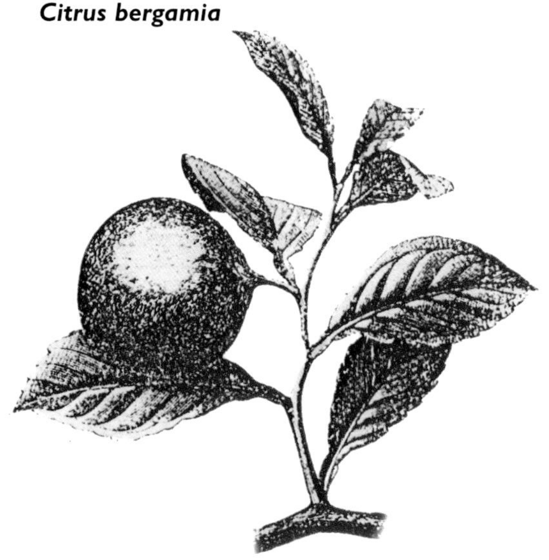

Bergamot is a small and very bitter orange. It is grown in Italy, where it has been used in traditional remedies for many years.

Plant profile: bergamot is a small bitter orange grown in the Lombardy region of Italy near the town of Bergamo. The fruit has long been used in the traditional medicine of the area as a remedy for fevers and low immunity. The essential oil from the peel is best known as the flavoring of Earl Grey tea, giving the drink a fresh, citrusy flavor.

Safety information: bergamot is strongly phototoxic; avoid exposing the skin to strong sunlight or sunbeds for at least 12 hours after application. FCF (furano-coumarin free) bergamot oil is available with the phototoxic constituent removed, but the aroma of the oil is much reduced.

Fragrance profile: fresh, bright, citrusy, and sweet, developing softer, rounder, and warmer tones later.

Main uses: boosts immunity, helps to combat colds, influenza, and respiratory complaints; eases the symptoms of vaginal thrush; soothes anxiety, depression, helps to lift low spirits, and combat stress.

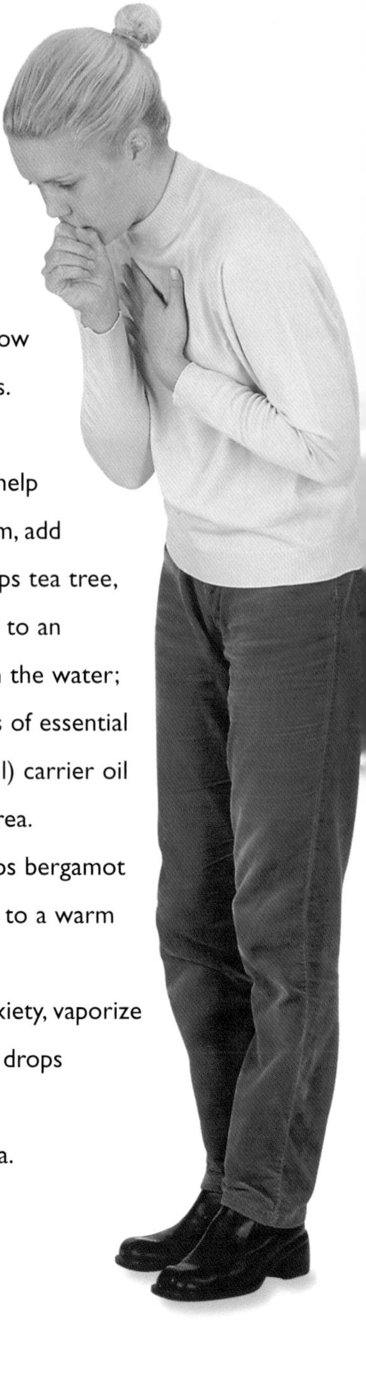

Suggested blends: to help boost the immune system, add 2 drops bergamot, 2 drops tea tree, and 1 drop black pepper to an evening bath and relax in the water; then add the same drops of essential oil to 2 teaspoons (10 ml) carrier oil and massage the chest area.

For thrush, add 2 drops bergamot and 3 drops sandalwood to a warm bath to soothe the area.

To ease stress and anxiety, vaporize 3 drops bergamot and 3 drops frankincense to create a warm and uplifting aroma.

Bergamot and tea tree oils help to improve general immunity.

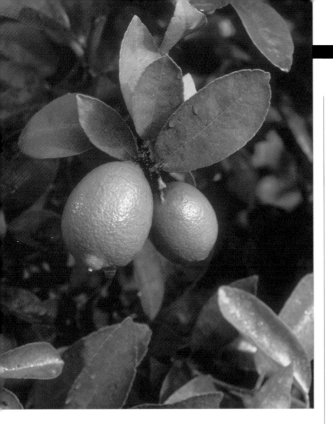

Fresh green limes are popular in Caribbean cooking. They are also an excellent source of vitamin C.

Lime

Citrus aurantifolia

Plant profile: an evergreen citrus tree, this is thorny with smooth aromatic leaves and small white flowers which turn into the fruits. Limes are about half the size of lemons and are a rich green in color. Limes are an excellent source of vitamin C and are widely used in cookery recipes from the West Indies. The oil is expressed from the peel. The main centers of production are Florida, Cuba, and Central America.

Safety information: lime is moderately phototoxic; you should avoid exposing the skin to strong sunlight or a sunbed for at least 12 hours after application.

Fragrance profile: bitter, green, and fresh with a powerful zest and sharp fruity notes.

Main uses: helps detoxify and improve areas of cellulite; eases chest infections, respiratory complaints, and catarrh; clears the head and improves concentration.

Suggested blends: to detoxify, use a skin brush to stimulate the circulation, then add 2 drops lime, 3 drops juniper, and 5 drops cypress to 4 teaspoons (20 ml) carrier oil and massage affected areas, as an evening treatment.

To relieve respiratory complaints, add 3 drops lime and 3 drops eucalyptus to a large bowl of nearly boiling water and inhale the vapors, twice daily for 20 minutes.

To clear the head, increase alertness, and improve the atmosphere in stuffy rooms, vaporize 3 drops lime and 3 drops peppermint.

Vaporize a mixture of peppermint and lime essential oils to help improve concentration.

Simple Essential Oil Skincare

Essential oils can be used as the basis of a simple and effective skincare routine. They are particularly effective when used at night, because lying horizontally promotes an excellent supply of blood to your face for maximum absorption of essential oils through the skin. Use the chart below to identify your skin type and choose the blends that will be most suitable for you.

Skin types

Normal—smooth and supple, clear in appearance, fine-textured
Dry—dull-textured, dehydrated, tends to tighten up in wind or warm temperatures
Mature—evident expression lines and slackness around eyes and mouth, less elasticity
Oily—shiny, with large obvious pores, tendency to blemishes
Combination—a greasy patch over forehead, nose, and chin; dry cheek areas
Sensitive—often very pale, sensitive to sunlight and cosmetics, allergic tendency

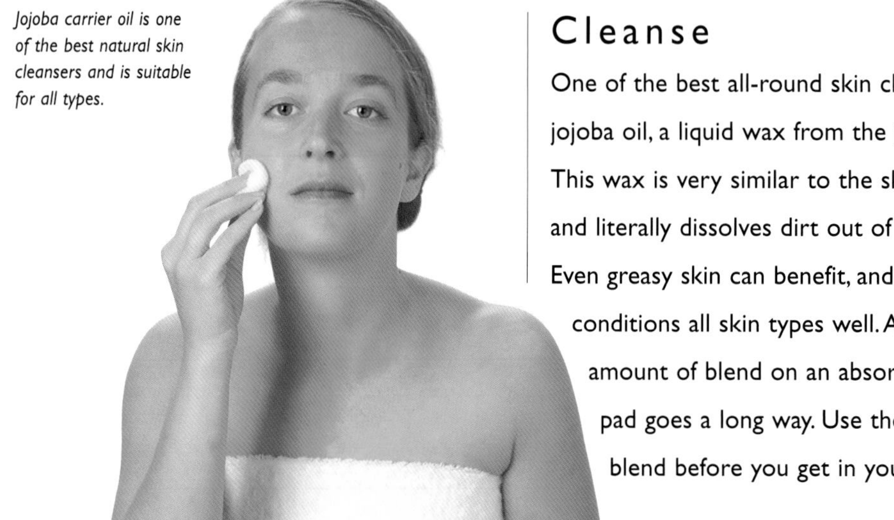

Jojoba carrier oil is one of the best natural skin cleansers and is suitable for all types.

Cleanse

One of the best all-round skin cleansers is jojoba oil, a liquid wax from the jojoba bean. This wax is very similar to the skin's own oils, and literally dissolves dirt out of the pores. Even greasy skin can benefit, and jojoba conditions all skin types well. A small amount of blend on an absorbent cotton pad goes a long way. Use the cleansing blend before you get in your bath, so the steam from the bath can further open the pores before you use your toner.

Add one of the following blends to 4 teaspoons (20 ml) jojoba oil:

Normal/dry/mature skin: 2 drops frankincense, 4 drops sandalwood, 4 drops orange.
Oily/combination skin: 2 drops juniper, 3 drops cypress, 5 drops lemon.
Sensitive skin (half the proportions): 2 drops roman camomile, 3 drops lavender.

These blends should be used within 4 weeks. They can be kept in the fridge or at room temperature. (They last longer in the fridge.)

Tone

Good drug stores and essential oil suppliers sell floral waters, the by-products of the distillation process, which make very good toners. Use a small amount on an absorbent cotton pad to freshen the skin before the moisturizing treatment. The following flower waters are recommended:

Normal/dry/mature skin: pure rose water or pure neroli water.

Floral waters make very gentle skin toners. Good drug stores will stock them.

Oily/combination skin: pure lavender water.
Sensitive skin: pure camomile water or pure rose water.
Floral waters will last up to six months if kept in the fridge.

Moisturize

Night time facial treatment oils have a shelf life of about four weeks and can be made up either in sweet almond oil, recommended for dry or mature skins, or jojoba, for all skin types.

Add to 4 teaspoons (20 ml) of carrier oil:

Normal/dry/mature skin: 2 drops rose, 3 drops neroli, 5 drops frankincense.
Oily/combination skin: 3 drops geranium, 3 drops cypress, 4 drops lemon.
Sensitive skin (half proportions): 3 drops roman camomile, 2 drops rose.

Massage a small amount into your face for 10 minutes, using upward strokes on your cheeks and tiny circles around your eye sockets and over your forehead. Be careful not to wipe the blend into your eyes.

Special Massage Blends

Here are some special massage blends for you to try, for physical, mood-related, and seasonal reasons. They are all designed to be made up in 4 teaspoons (20 ml) carrier oil, such as sweet almond, jojoba, or grapeseed, a lighter and less greasy base oil. They all have a four-week shelf life. Massage relevant areas gently, using relaxing sweeping movements. Sometimes you may wish to work on yourself, but it can be soothing to let someone else—a close friend or partner—massage you.

Physical Tonics

Here are four blends for hard-working areas of the body which are constantly under strain.

Super muscle tone: for sports massage to energize and strengthen the muscles—4 drops rosemary, 2 drops lemongrass, and 4 drops ginger.

Barefoot bliss: a massage blend to help cool and soothe tired and aching feet after a long day—3 drops peppermint, 3 drops black pepper, and 4 drops lavender.

Chest relief: a wonderful blend for a chest massage to ease respiratory problems—

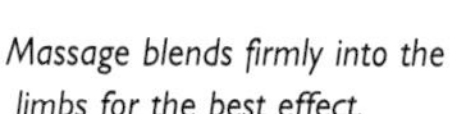

Massage blends firmly into the limbs for the best effect.

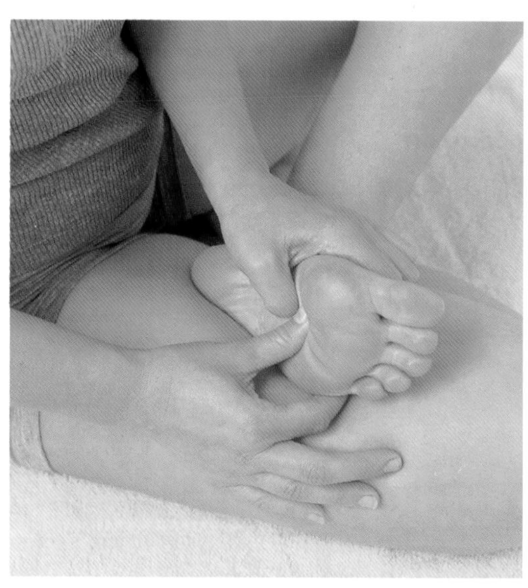

A foot massage warms and relaxes tired feet. It feels even better if someone else does it for you!

3 drops cedarwood, 3 drops frankincense, and 4 drops lemon.

Neck and shoulder rescue: ask a friend or your partner to massage this blend into your aching muscles—2 drops vetiver, 3 drops ginger, and 5 drops lavender.

Mood Mixtures

Here are some ideas for more subtle blends with rich aromas. You will find them useful for lifting the spirits and easing emotional stresses and strains.

Beat the blues: 3 drops orange, 4 drops grapefruit, and 3 drops sandalwood makes a wonderful relaxing, uplifting, and de-stressing blend for massage.

PMT reviver: at that low time in your monthly cycle, try a blend of 4 drops palmarosa, 2 drops patchouli, and 4 drops bergamot for an evening massage blend.

On cloud nine: when you need to escape and have no cares in the world, try 4 drops grapefruit, 2 drops neroli, and 4 drops cardamom for a dreamy aroma.

Tropical retreat: create an exotic mood with 2 drops ylang ylang, 4 drops mandarin, and 4 drops sandalwood—this is a fruity, rich, and floral feast for the senses.

Seasonal Treats

As your energies vary, you may find that you need different massage blends to pick you up at different times of the year. Massage is particularly effective after a bath, as the skin absorbs the blend better. Spending time being massaged also helps improve your sleep—when you rest like this, your whole body can restore itself and your mind can be at peace.

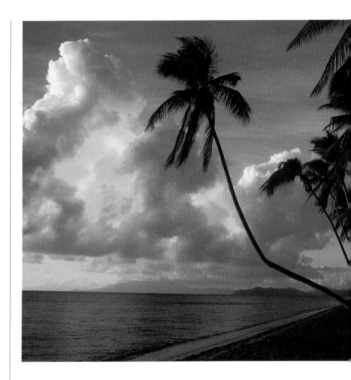

Inhale the aromas of the oils in the blends and float off into your own haven of tranquility—a tropical beach, for example.

Springtime freshener: to help to revitalize and energize you after the long drag of wintertime—4 drops lemon, 3 drops juniper, and 3 drops peppermint.

Summer skin food: use the following blend in 4 teaspoons (20 ml) jojoba oil to nourish the skin deeply—3 drops sandalwood, 2 drops patchouli, and 5 drops frankincense.

Fall spiritual reviver: to uplift you as the nights draw in—4 drops mandarin, 3 drops may chang, and 3 drops coriander.

Winter energizer: for aches, stiffness, and low vitality—2 drops vetiver, 3 drops lemongrass, and 5 drops nutmeg.

Essential Oils in Everyday Life

Essential oils are a wonderful and natural way to keep your environment fresh and to raise your energy levels. They are very portable and can easily be adapted to suit different locations and needs. Here are some ideas for using oils simply and effectively.

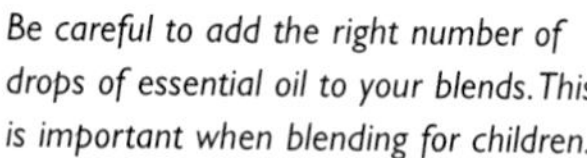

Be careful to add the right number of drops of essential oil to your blends. This is important when blending for children.

Home

In your home, essential oils help to personalize your living space.

Kitchen

This is one of the most frequently used and also most potentially accident-prone areas. Always keep lavender and tea tree to hand—you can use either oil neat for cuts, burns, scalds, and other mishaps (put 2 drops on an absorbent cotton pad).

A kitchen spray to remove stale odors and freshen counters can be made in a pump-action spray bottle filled with a scant ½ cup/100 ml water, 10 drops peppermint, and 15 drops lemon. Shake the bottle and spray mist into the air, or spray counters and wipe them down.

A pump-action spray bottle helps to spread essential oils over a much wider area.

Dining room

A vaporizer adds atmosphere to a dinner party. For example, a festive gathering can be fragranced with 3 drops mandarin and 3 drops nutmeg, or a summer party with 3 drops may chang and 3 drops orange. One dose of essential oils in a vaporizer will last up to 2 hours.

Living room

Again, a vaporizer can clear the atmosphere, neutralize pet odors, and freshen the air. A combination like 3 drops tea tree and 3 drops lemon helps if someone has a cold or influenza. After a party the night before, 3 drops peppermint and 3 drops rosemary is very uplifting and refreshing.

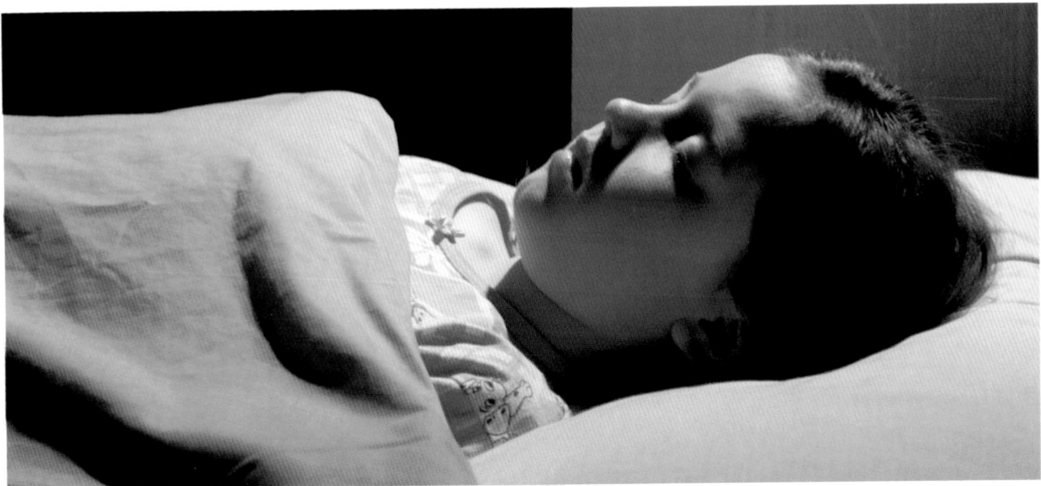

Vaporizing oils in a bedroom will improve the quality of sleep and scent the room delightfully as well.

Child's bedroom

An electric vaporizer is recommended for safety reasons. Essential oils can really help sleep. Add 3 drops lavender and 3 drops orange for a soothing aroma; or 3 drops lavender and 3 drops eucalyptus if there are chest problems. Try to start the vaporizer at least 10 minutes before your child goes to bed—this spreads the fragrance into the room as they fall asleep.

Travel

Essential oils can help you on the move.

Car

Vaporizers are available that plug into the cigarette lighter socket, or you can put oils on a tissue. On long journeys, 3 drops peppermint and 3 drops rosemary will help you stay alert.

Keep a tissue in your pocket when you're traveling on long journeys—you can inhale oils from it when you have a break.

Trains and airplanes

Carry one or two essential oils with you and put a few drops onto a tissue to inhale. Lavender will help you relax, peppermint and rosemary will wake you up, and lemon or tea tree will help ease sinus congestion.

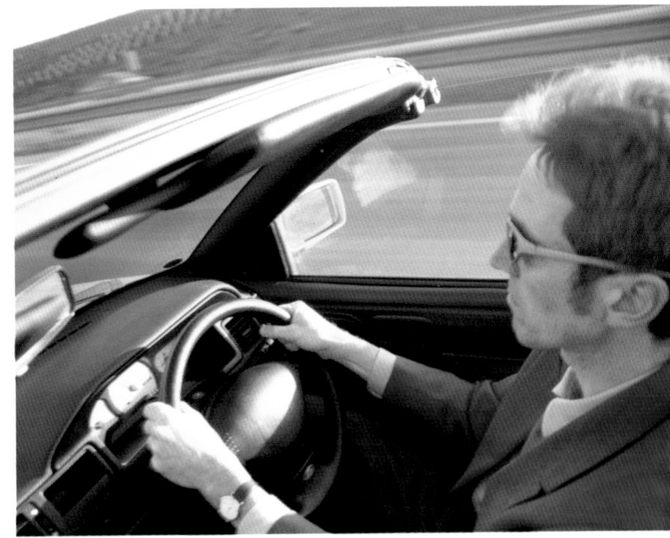

Buying and Storing Essential Oils

Here are some simple guidelines to follow to help you get the best out of your essential oil collection.

Buying Oils

There are many essential oil suppliers now selling to the public, and there is, unfortunately, a huge variation in the quality and therapeutic effectiveness of the oils available. True essential oils are not just a manufactured product, they are produced year by year and harvests can be affected by many environmental changes. Cheap essential oils are much more likely to be synthetic copies than the genuine article. Check that your supplier sources oils directly from growers.

You need to buy your oils in dark glass bottles to protect them from UV light. Oils should also have a drop dispenser in the neck of the bottle to release one drop at a time to help you calculate your blends. This is also an important safety feature: open-necked bottles are a risk to children, who may swallow the contents. In any case, keep all essential oils well out of children's reach.

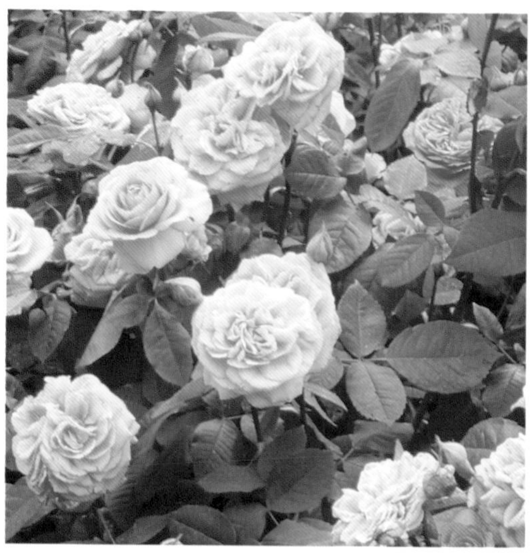

Many plants are expensive to harvest and these oils can be costly to buy. However, their divine scent makes it all worthwhile!

Storing Oils

Essential oils degrade with time. Their constituents oxidize and become unstable, smelling rancid. The cooler and more tightly closed they are kept, the longer the shelf life. How long you keep your oils depends on the storage temperature: in the fridge, most oils last up to two years, citrus oils one year.

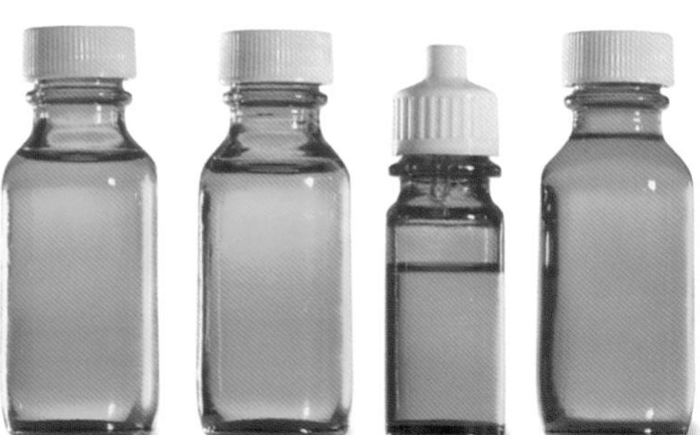

Dark glass bottles with integrated stoppers or drop dispensers are vital if you are planning to use a lot of essential oils.

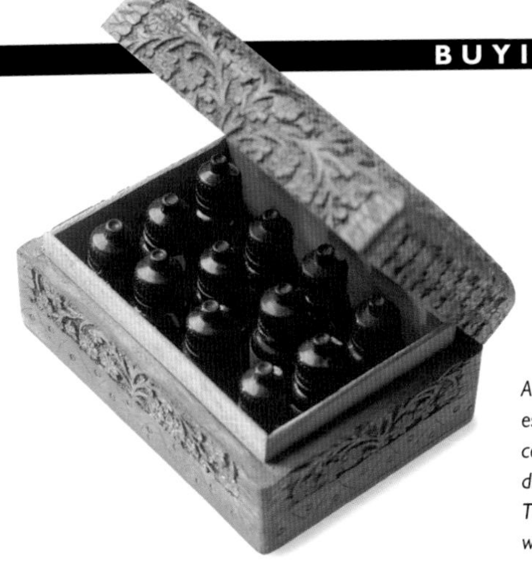

Always keep essential oils cool and out of direct sunlight. They also keep well in the fridge.

At room temperature, most oils last up to one year, citrus oils six months. The shelf life is calculated from the first day you open a new bottle. Write a date on the label or place a sticker on the bottle to remind you of the use-by date. If you are keeping oils in the fridge, you are advised to put them in an airtight box first to stop the fragrances spreading to your milk and dairy products! Out of the fridge, keep the oils tightly closed, in the dark, and in a cool place. Do not use essential oils once they have gone past their shelf life, because they are then more likely to cause skin reactions.

Keeping essential oils in the fridge extends their shelf life. Make sure that the bottles are airtight at all times.

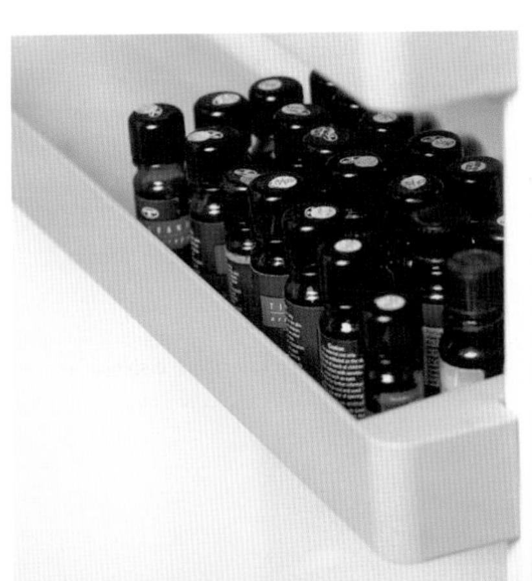

Recommended Suppliers

The following suppliers do mail order and sell high-quality ranges of essential oils.

Aromatherapy Products Ltd (suppliers of the Tisserand range, selling to 30 countries)
Newtown Road, Hove, East Sussex
BN3 7BA, UK
Tel: +44 (0)1273 325666;
Fax: +44 (0)1273 208444
Call them for your nearest stockist or mail order enquiries.

Essentially Oils Ltd
8–10 Mount Farm, Junction Road, Chipping Norton, Oxfordshire OX7 6NP, UK
Tel: +44 (0)1608 659544;
Fax: +44 (0)1608 659566
www.essentiallyoils.com
email: sales@essentiallyoils.com
Mail order enquiries welcome.

In the USA you are recommended to contact **National Association for Holistic Aromatherapy (NAHA)** for details of suppliers: 2000 2nd Avenue, Suite 206, Seattle WA 98121, USA
Tel: +001 (206) 2560741
www.naha.org

Glossary

Camphoraceous note
a medicinal and sharp aroma, such as marjoram.

Carrier oil
a vegetable oil used to dilute essential oils.

Cellulite
waterlogged fatty tissue deposits, particularly on thighs.

Citrus note
fresh and fruity aroma like citrus fruit.

Constituent
a fragrance ingredient of an essential oil (most oils contain up to 150).

Detoxifying
assists in the removal of toxins from the system.

Distillation
extraction of essential oils through steam followed by condensation.

Drop dispenser
a mechanism in the neck of a bottle to dispense one drop of oil.

Expression
pressing essential oils out of citrus fruit peel.

Floral note
a sweet flowery fragrance, such as rose.

Floral water
the by-product of distillation, delicately fragranced, very mild on the skin.

Inhalation
breathing in essential oil molecules to clear the chest.

Photosynthesis
plant process of sugar production using sunlight.

Phototoxic
causing skin reactions in sunlight.

Pungent note
a warm and sometimes spicy aroma.

Sensitive skin
delicate, allergy-prone skin with a tendency to rashes.

Shelf life
the length of time an essential oil can be kept before it degrades.

Solvent extraction
fragrance extraction using chemical solvents.

Synthetic fragrance
an aroma created by artificial chemicals.

Vaporizer
a unit designed to spread the fragrance of essential oils into a room.

Useful Addresses and Websites

United Kingdom

International Federation of Aromatherapists (IFA)
Stamford House, 2/4 Chiswick High Road,
London W4 1TH, UK
Tel: +44 (0)20 8742 2605

International Society of Professional Aromatherapists (ISPA)
ISPA House, 82 Ashby Road, Hinckley,
Leicestershire LE10 1SN, UK
Tel: +44 (0)1455 637987

Register of Qualified Aromatherapists (RQA)
PO BOX 3431, Danbury, Chelmsford, Essex
CM3 4UA, UK

N.B. In 2002, these three organizations are intending to amalgamate as one body called the International Federation of Professional Aromatherapists (IFPA).

USA

American Alliance of Aromatherapy
PO BOX 750428, Petaluma, CA 94975, USA
Tel: +001 (707) 778 6762

National Association for Holistic Aromatherapy (NAHA)
2000 2nd Avenue, Suite 206, Seattle WA 98121
USA
Tel: +001 (206) 265 0741
www.naha.org

Australia

International Federation of Aromatherapists
PO Box 2210, Central Park, Victoria 3145,
Australia
Tel. +0061 1902 240 125

Index